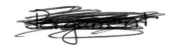

D1571181

DAY TREATMENT FOR CHILDREN WITH EMOTIONAL DISORDERS

Volume 1

A Model in Action

DAY TREATMENT FOR CHILDREN WITH EMOTIONAL DISORDERS
Volume 1
A Model in Action

Edited by
Sara Goodman Zimet
and
Gordon K. Farley

University of Colorado Health Sciences Center
Denver, Colorado

PLENUM PRESS • NEW YORK AND LONDON

Library of Congress Cataloging-in-Publication Data

Day treatment for children with emotional disorders / edited by Sara
 Goodman Zimet and Gordon K. Farley.
      p.   cm.
   Includes bibliographical references and index.
   Contents: v. 1. A Model in action.
   ISBN 0-306-43743-0 (v. 1)
   1. Psychiatric day treatment for children--United States.
 I. Zimet, Sara Goodman.   II. Farley, Gordon K.
   [DNLM: 1. Affective Disorders--in infancy & childhood.
 2. Affective Disorders--therapy. 3. Day Care--in infancy &
 childhood. 4. Day Care--organization & administration.   WS 350.6
 D275]
 RJ504.53.D38 1991
 618.92'89--dc20
 DNLM/DLC
 for Library of Congress   91-2086
                                                               CIP

ISBN 0-306-43743-0

© 1991 Plenum Press, New York
A Division of Plenum Publishing Corporation
233 Spring Street, New York, N.Y. 10013

Printed in the United States of America

Dedicated to my husband, Carl;
and to my children, Greg, Andy,
Lynne, and Flo.

—SGZ

Dedicated to my wife, Kiki;
my sons, Steven and David;
my mother, Neva; my brothers, Curtis and Robert;
and my sister, Patricia.

—GKF

Contributors

Nanci Avitable, 2833 South Wabash Circle, Denver, Colorado 80231

Caroline L. Corkey, the Day Care Center, Department of Psychiatry, University of Colorado Health Sciences Center, Denver, Colorado 80262

Charles A. Ekanger, the Day Care Center, Department of Psychiatry, University of Colorado Health Sciences Center, Denver, Colorado 80262

Gordon K. Farley, the Day Care Center, Department of Psychiatry, University of Colorado Health Sciences Center, Denver, Colorado 80262

Ralph Imhoff, the Day Care Center, Department of Psychiatry, University of Colorado Health Sciences Center, Denver, Colorado 80262

John A. Kayser, Graduate School of Social Work, University of Denver, Denver, Colorado 80208

Carol L. Lee, the Day Care Center, Department of Psychiatry, University of Colorado Health Sciences Center, Denver, Colorado 80262

Patricia Mulligan, the Day Care Center, Department of Psychiatry, University of Colorado Health Sciences Center, Denver, Colorado 80262

Phyllis C. Parsons, the Day Care Center, Department of Psychiatry, University of Colorado Health Sciences Center, Denver, Colorado 80262

Geraldine F. Schultz, the Day Care Center, Department of Psychiatry, University of Colorado Health Sciences Center, Denver, Colorado 80262

Abe E. Tenorio, the Day Care Center, Department of Psychiatry, University of Colorado Health Sciences Center, Denver, Colorado 80262

Sara Goodman Zimet, the Day Care Center, Department of Psychiatry, University of Colorado Health Sciences Center, Denver, Colorado 80262

Preface

The life span of day treatment for children in the United States is relatively short, covering a period of about 50 years. Although the first 20 years saw little growth in the number of centers operating around the country, the concept of day treatment was recognized by the Joint Commission on Mental Illness and Health in 1961 as the most significant treatment innovation of this century. Enthusiasm for this treatment modality gained impetus from growing dissatisfaction among many mental health care providers who had no choice but to place children in a highly restrictive hospital environment. Day treatment did not carry the stigma associated with inpatient placement. The children could now remain with their own families and within their own communities. The parents could be actively included in their child's treatment. This new modality avoided the short- and long-term negative effects of institutionalization, and there was a favorable cost discrepancy between day and inpatient mental health services. In more recent years, there has been growing evidence of the efficacy of day treatment as an intensive therapeutic environment for children and their parents. Despite these advantages, day treatment has continued to be underutilized in favor of inpatient treatment by both the psychiatric community and third-party payers. Only recently is it being acknowledged by some insurers as a therapeutically sound and financially advantageous alternative to inpatient services. Consequently, it is showing signs of intense growth nationally.

In order to meet the demands for day treatment mental health services, we need answers to questions regarding the "nuts and bolts" of starting up a center; we need to review the wisdom gained by centers that have been operating programs successfully; we need to consider the range of choices in theoretical models and in treatment components. It is the purpose of the two volumes comprising *Day Treatment for Children with Emotional Disorders* to present this information to both the novice and experienced practitioner and to the academician.

In Volume 1, *A Model in Action,* we have examined the salient features of an actual program that has been operating since 1962—the Day Care Center. It is located within the Division of Child Psychiatry, Department of Psychiatry, of the University of Colorado Health Sciences Center. The primary focus of the chapters in this volume is the personal and practical issues of operating this program. We have presented the reader with a clinical case study of our program by describing its various components and the forces from within and from without that bear upon its day-to-day functioning. The volume is organized around four parts. The first part is introductory. The second part focuses on our clinical and educational programs and includes nine chapters of detailed descriptions. Administrative issues are examined in two chapters in the third part. The three chapters in our concluding part concentrate on our research and program evaluation efforts.

In Volume 2, *Programs across the Country,* we have focused on both practical and theoretical issues in three parts. The first part consists of three chapters dealing with issues about starting up day treatment services. The second part includes six chapters, each describing a day treatment program from a different theoretical perspective. The final part, the Appendix, provides the reader with a comprehensive annotated bibliography of publications on day treatment for children with emotional disorders.

To those of our readers who are interested in learning about day treatment in Western Europe, we would like to refer them to two recent issues of the *International Journal of Partial Hospitalization* that were edited by us (1988, Volume 5, Numbers 1 and 2). They include descriptions of programs in England, France, The Netherlands, Norway, Sweden, Switzerland, and Germany. Five of the chapters are written by mental health professionals in those countries and six by Sara Goodman Zimet as a result of a fellowship she received from the World Rehabilitation Fund's International Exchange of Experts and Information in Rehabilitation. The fellowship was supported (in part) from a grant from the National Institute of Disability and Rehabilitation Research, U.S. Department of Education, Washington, DC 20201, Grant No. G008435012. Commentaries on each of the descriptions were made by Gordon K. Farley, who has been active in day psychiatric treatment and research for 23 years and has been director of the Day Care Center for over 17 years.

In the process of preparing these volumes, we realized that there are many terms in current use that describe the day treatment modality, such as *day hospital, partial hospital, psychoeducational, psychiatric day treat-*

ment, and so forth. Although our own center is located within a university health sciences center, we decided to use *day treatment* as the generic term that would apply to hospital-affiliated and nonaffiliated treatment programs. In making this choice, we have attempted to identify this treatment modality as existing within the child's and parents' community rather than within an institution separated from that community.

We would like to thank the children at the Day Care Center who contributed their illustrations to the two volumes comprising *Day Treatment for Children with Emotional Disorders.* These illustrations were done during their routine work with their art teacher (and head teacher), Ralph Imhoff. We are also indebted to Richard Simons, professor of psychiatry at the University of Colorado Health Sciences Center, for his helpful suggestions regarding our editorial role.

SARA GOODMAN ZIMET
GORDON K. FARLEY

Denver, Colorado

Contents

**Chapter 10. Special Projects in the Treatment Program: Their
Birth, Development, and Occasional Demise 143**

Phyllis C. Parsons and Ralph Imhoff

PART III. ADMINISTRATIVE ISSUES. 163

Sara Goodman Zimet, Gordon K. Farley, and Nanci Avitable

Sara Goodman Zimet and Gordon K. Farley

Caroline L. Corkey and Sara Goodman Zimet

I

Introduction

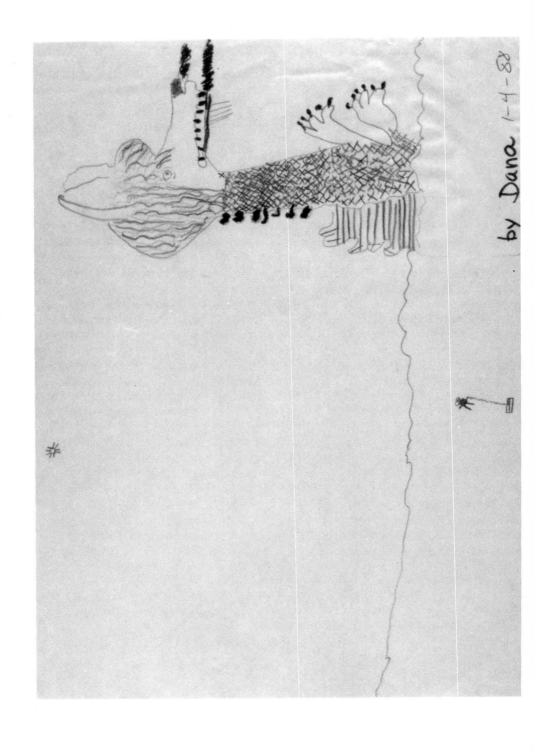

by Dana 1-4-88

In this introductory chapter, "A Profile of the Day Care Center, Past and Present," Gordon Farley orients the reader to the volume, *A Model in Action*. He places today's program at the Day Care Center within its historical context. He identifies the people and their beliefs as well as the societal forces that contributed to formulating the structure and orientation of the treatment program over its 28 years of existence. Here we have a developmental profile of a dynamic day treatment program. In describing the components of today's program, Gordon Farley, who has been the director of the Day Care Center since 1973, sets the stage for the chapters that follow in Parts II, III, and IV with their more detailed accounts of the many components of the clinical, educational, administrative, and research programs.

1

A Profile of the Day Care Center, Past and Present

GORDON K. FARLEY

INTRODUCTION

On the first day, or was it the eighth day, Eve spoke softly to Adam and said, "Adam, we are living in a time of transition." This tired, well-worn joke makes the obvious point that in a history of 28 years, an institution changes, adjusts, recoils, reels, agonizes, reappraises, and sometimes moves forward. As in human development, institutional development is not even but occurs in fits and starts and is marked by progress and regression and at times much lateral movement.

It is interesting to consider the central forces that influenced our development and to evaluate the resultant directions. In retrospect, it seems as though early developments were heavily influenced by conceptual and treatment innovations and creativity, and more recent developments have been more heavily influenced by fiscal exigencies, emergencies, and as our department administrator puts it, "financial realities" (of which clinicians are often woefully ignorant).

THE SIXTIES

In 1960, in the state of Colorado, state funds became available for the construction of a psychiatric facility for children. Gaston E. Blom,

GORDON K. FARLEY • The Day Care Center, Department of Psychiatry, University of Colorado Health Sciences Center, Denver, Colorado 80262.

the head of the Child Psychiatry Division, an adult and child psychoanalyst with remarkable foresight, decided that day treatment had educational, ethical, economic, and efficacy advantages over inpatient treatment. His wish was to combine information, research, and technical
advances from the fields of psychoanalysis, psychology, child development, education, and child psychiatry.

The doors opened in September 1962 with eight children in daily
attendance. From the beginning, the commitment was to the completion
of treatment rather than to a patch-up, short-term, way station to the
next treatment setting and the next approach. Classroom engineering
methods that included changing children's behavior through alterations
in or arrangement of the physical environment were an important part
of the professional orientation. A scientific view permeated the setting.
Ideas were to be judged on their observed merit and effectiveness rather
than on their closeness to an adhered-to theoretical ideal. Children's
behaviors were to be understood from a variety of perspectives including psychodynamic, learning theory, sociocultural, and others.

An architect, teachers, social workers, a cook, a driver, psychologists, and secretarial staff members were hired, and attempts were made
to put these principles into practice. One of the underlying views was
that communication problems occur among professionals because their
views of children's problems, including causative and maintaining influences, vary markedly. One way to overcome these divergent views was to
have one person (such as a psychiatrist) function in another person's role
(such as a teacher's). Thus we had teachers doing child psychotherapy,
child psychiatrists doing classroom teaching, and drivers doing group
therapy. These directions also were encouraged by the egalitarian, social
consciousness, indigenous mental health worker, community mental
health movements of the 1960s. There was a strong effort to apply
psychoanalytic concepts to the classroom situation. Psychoanalytically
oriented supervision was given for teachers and the social work staff.
The focus in these sessions was on the transference and countertransfer-
ence aspects of working with disturbed children. Many of the professional staff members were involved in a personal psychoanalysis or psychoanalytically oriented psychotherapy. Psychoanalytic thinking was
applied to such items as classroom seating arrangements and teacher
and student mobility in the classroom. It was decided that children
should remain seated at double desks and that the teacher should approach the students, sit with them, and teach them. The classrooms were
built to accommodate 12 students in each one, and team teaching, with
two teachers working together with different groups of students in the
same classroom, was applied.

In retrospect, it is remarkable how unfettered we were by financial constraints. We admitted children and families who seemed to have some interest in changing, some motivation for treatment, some commitment to the treatment process, and some psychological mindedness. Ability to pay for treatment seldom was considered in the equation.

Group problem solving was the method of resolution of disputes and disagreements among staff members about treatment philosophy and other matters.

After 1 year of functioning with an interim director at the Day Care Center, Gaston Blom stepped down from his position as head of the child psychiatry division and assumed the leadership of the center. One of the organizing ideas was that things would be learned in this small, restricted, controlled, highly observable setting and then these principles could be applied to help emotionally disturbed and learning-disabled children in public school settings.

Community involvement was a significant part of the Day Care Center activities. Community psychiatry was growing rapidly, stimulated by the Mental Health Acts of 1963 and 1965, and public schools were seen as offering open arms to psychiatric–psychological input. In addition, many of our consultation services were given without cost to several of the local large and small school districts, headstart centers, and anyone else who would stand still for the experience. Schools, at this time, were dealing with racial integration, early childhood intervention programs, and recently mandated special education programs. The Day Care Center staff felt that this was a perfect time to bring psychiatric knowledge to educational settings. Social changes, including increased attention to racism and sexism in textbooks and the larger society, had an impact on our program and were frequent topics of intense discussion. Multiracial readers were introduced into our classrooms, and we became very aware of the racial–ethnic mix of both our patient population and our staff. Unconscious racism on an individual and societal level was openly discussed.

Family therapy and family-therapy approaches were enthusiastically applied, and visits to patients' homes, both for evaluation and treatment, became common (see the chapter by Ekanger).

Information from learning disabilities research was important for a time. A view of auditory and visual processing and materials intended to repair these learning deficits were very much in evidence in our setting during the late 1960s.

The psycholinguistic learning disabilities model of Kirk and Kirk (1971) influenced our educational program. Language processing was thought of as a chain of events, and treatment was supposed to focus on the weakest links in the chain through the use of developmental learning materials. Brain injury and learning disabilities were widely discussed (Cruickshank, Bentzen, Ratzeburg, & Tannhauser, 1961; Cruickshank, 1966).

Psychomotor training programs based on the work of Newel Kephart (1964), Bryant Cratty (1969, 1970), and others were applied. Visuomotor training based on the work of Marianne Frostig (1970) and Jean Ayres's (1973) sensory integration therapy were heavily used.

ON INTO THE SEVENTIES

This period of frenetic activity and theoretical foment took place over a 10-year period. In 1971, the leadership of the Day Care Center was turned over to Mark Rudnick, a clinical child psychologist and psychoanalyst in training. A new emphasis was brought to bear on individual child psychotherapeutic work. Individual child psychotherapy sessions were microscopically examined through the use of videotaped segments. There was particular interest in parent-loss and the subsequent effects on personality development. Special treatment efforts designed to ameliorate the negative effects of this experience were introduced. This era was ended abruptly by the untimely death of Mark Rudnick in December 1973.

The next era was one that focused on designing and implementing a standard data base, program evaluation, and revision of our educational program (see the chapters on establishing a data base and on our educational program). Gordon Farley became the center's director and Sara Zimet the director of research and program evaluation.

In June 1975, a preliminary examination of the records of our child graduates indicated that, in addition to minimal gains made in their academic performance, low motivation for learning was characteristic of these youngsters. In order to define a new educational approach that would maximize the academic and behavioral growth of our students, we took a closer look at the problems associated with their learning in school, identified aspects of the program that related to these problems, and proposed certain interventions. In examining the interventions recommended, it became apparent that they closely matched the integrated curriculum model. The previous educational model emphasized age and grade norms of performance in separately taught subject areas, using traditional texts and workbooks. Most of the work was concerned with remediation of academic deficits; thus curriculum experiences were skill oriented rather than topic oriented. Training was provided in improving

perceptual-motor skills through exercises and games, and special training was given in problem solving through simulation. All curriculum decisions and choices were made by the teachers and handed down to the
students.

By adopting the integrated curriculum, a significant shift occurred.
A non-age/grade curriculum characterized this model, where each child
was accepted at whatever instructional level he or she was operating, and
each was provided with learning experiences based on his or her interests and abilities. Children became involved in making choices concerning topics to study, activities to perform, and materials to be used.
Plans were devised with the teacher and individual plan books kept by
the children. Teachers acted as resource persons who encouraged and
influenced the direction and growth of learning. Clear expectations that
responsibility for learning was jointly shared by teachers and students
was maintained.

While working on these self-selected areas of interest, refinement of
skills occurred under the teacher's guidance, and the rationale for
"school learning" became evident. Firsthand, concrete experiences such
as field trips, follow-up discussions, exploratory work with different
kinds of materials, and opportunities to play out and dramatize or make
some other representation of the experiences and explore their mean-
ings in depth were critical characteristics of the program. Resources
from the community were used extensively. Parents also were viewed as
part of the talent bank. Resource centers within the school for math,
language experiences, crafts, drama, and the like provided other opportunities for children to explore interests in greater depth and practice
the skills they needed to develop.

The children were given feedback on their test performance and on
their daily work in school. The latter was accomplished through peer
evaluation groups led by the teachers and from individual interactions
between all staff members and the children. Self-evaluation was also part
of the process of the records kept by each student. For example, in their
planning books, they were required to evaluate the outcome of their
plans and to base the next step of their plan on the evaluation they had
made. Problems, as they arose in and out of the classroom were also used
as a vehicle for increasing their problem-solving repertoires. Students
were encouraged to formulate and use different approaches and to evaluate the effectiveness of their strategies. Group discussions were also
structured around making hypotheses and checking them out. For example, in a group project on rocketry, the children guessed what kinds
of things would occur when their rockets were launched. They observed
the actual operation and later discussed it in terms of their own expecta-

tions and the reasons there were discrepancies. Through a crisis control system (see chapter on Standby by Farley), problems requiring the intervention of a neutral party were dealt with in a similar fashion.

Remediation of cognitive, perceptual-motor, language, and social skills was carried out primarily within this same program structure. For example, fine and gross motor coordination was practiced through crafts and athletic activities rather than through the use of exercises out of their life context. However, where more intense remediation was called for, remedial therapists worked with the children individually.

Thus an interdisciplinary integrated approach to understanding the children and planning educational and psychotherapeutic interventions was complemented by the integrated curriculum program.

Our romance with the integrated curriculum was torrid and intense. We immersed ourselves in the program, read books, had workshops, hired outside consultants and searched, discussed, and refined our ideas and plans during frequent retreats. Some staff members loved the integrated curriculum, and some hated it, but all of us were profoundly affected by it. Particularly when we first began the program, there was a great deal of resistance and apprehension. The question seemed to be whether we could control the children in what appeared to be such a loosely structured environment. Although there were many anecdotal data indicating the effectiveness of this approach, in our setting it proved too difficult to use without significant modifications. We attempted to adapt the curriculum by making adjustment for our children's need for structure and predictability and for their deficient academic skills. We never formally ended the plan, but various teachers gradually drifted more and more away from it and organized their own behaviorally oriented classroom, whole language approach classroom, or variations on these models. We learned a great deal from the experiment, and many residuals of the integrated curriculum still continue in our program today (please see the chapters on projects in the classroom and on the educational program).

From the research standpoint, our attention turned to evaluating certain aspects of the program and our clinical population (please see the chapter, "The Day Treatment Center as a Research Setting").

MOVING INTO THE EIGHTIES

Starting in about 1980, generating clinical fees became more and more important. Over a period of approximately 8 years, we have been required to move from generating about 10% of our total operating budget to now generating about 80% of it. This has had a profound effect on the length of treatment offered, the patient mix, and the general feelings of urgency of keeping our census high.

Our Philosophy of Treatment

We consider ourselves to be a developmentally oriented bio-psychosocial treatment program. We use a variety of approaches including those that can be termed *empirical, eclectic, family, systemic, strategic, psychodynamic, interpersonal, cognitive, motivational, rational,* and *learning theory* based. We also believe that a clinical research project is better than intuition or blind faith for answering a question about the effectiveness of a treatment model.

We always stay alert to the possibility of important biological contributors to psychiatric illness in children. In particular, we consider the possibilities of attention-deficit hyperactivity disorder, childhood major depression, early onset bipolar disorder, panic disorder, Tourette's syndrome, sleep disorders, and other childhood disorders with striking biological components. We attend carefully to the general physical health and nutrition of our children (please see the chapter on our food program by Zimet & Schultz). About one-half of our children have a trial of psychoactive medication. Medications that we have prescribed include psychostimulants, neuroleptics, antidepressants, anticonvulsants, Beta blockers, benzodiazepines, and anticonvulsants. Table 1 illustrates the way in which we gather biological, educational, psychological, and sociocultural information and apply treatments in these same domains.

Our Child Population

Many of the children we treat have physical illnesses that coexist with their psychiatric disorders. We have seen illnesses such as sickle cell disease, end stage renal failure, convulsive disorders, asthma, fragile X, Turner's syndrome, Tourette's syndrome, Down's syndrome, Noonan's syndrome, seropositivity for H.I.V., and hemophilia in our population. It has been our impression that our children have had more frequent physical illness than would be expected in a group of normal children. Prior to coming to our center, their illnesses have resulted in frequent school absences. In many cases, these illnesses and absences have contributed to academic underachievement and poor social relationships. Most often, in our program, however, their attendance markedly improves.

Undergirding our willingness to utilize many forms of treatment

Table 1. Evaluation and Treatment of the Day Patient

| | Sources of information | | |
| | Present | Past | |
	Descriptive	Developmental genetic	Treatment
Biological	Physical exam Laboratory tests Diagnostic pro- cedures	History of genetic and other constitutional factors History of physical ill- ness, injuries, opera- tions, abuse, and medications	Psychoactive medication Medication for phys- ical illnesses Somatic therapies Other medical treat- ments
Psychological	Mental status exam Psychological assessment Applied behavioral analysis Home behavior checklists	Developmental factors and experiences in infancy, childhood, adolescence, and adulthood	Individual psycho- dynamic child psychotherapy Individual parent psychotherapy Group child psychotherapy Family therapy Behavior modifica- tion programs Parent groups
Educational	Achievement testing School behavior checklists Classroom observations Perceptual-motor evaluations	Educational history	Milieu Educational programming Special education techniques Developmental learning materials Integrated curriculum Speech and language therapies
Sociocultural	Social support assessment Psychosocial stressor assessment	Family history Racial, religious, cul- tural, and so- cioeconomic background	Enhancing social supports Employment assistance Financial counseling

are some beliefs about what helps children and families to change and what helps to promote healthy growth and development.

We feel that the most important formative influence on children is intensive and long-term human relationships. Because relationships with all staff members are believed to be important in the emotional cure and growth of the children, we strive to have a stable staff in all areas of the milieu. It is our intention that these staff members are consistent, encouraging, supportive, warm, empathic, nurturant, and highly competent and will serve as models for growth. Our current special education teachers have a mean length of employment with us of 7.2 years. The director has been here for 22 years, the cook for 21 years, the chief social worker for 23 years, the educational psychologist for 17 years, and the social work staff for an average of about 10 years. Although we are a training facility, whenever possible we assign therapists for the duration of the time that the child is in day treatment. This emphasis on interpersonal relationships has roots in the psychoanalytic theory of identification and in the learning and cognitive theories of imitation.

We feel that children are more likely to learn to cope effectively with the problems they encounter in their natural environment under the following conditions:

1. The family system is engaged in the therapeutic experience. To this end, we offer child therapy and parent therapy. Individual and/or group psychotherapy is scheduled twice a week for children. Additionally, specifically designed behavior management programs aimed at helping children who may lose control in the group and who may require emergency interventions are available. A variety of therapeutic interventions also are offered to the children's caretakers on a once-a-week basis of both conflict-resolving and knowledge-imparting types. Many parents lack specific parenting skills, have had poor parental models themselves, and have sparse information regarding the range of appropriate techniques for rearing children. Our aim is to help them with conflicts that impair or impede their ability to offer authoritative, responsive, empathic parenting and a safe environment for the family. Both individual and group settings are offered, and negotiation regarding preferred modes of treatment is conducted.
2. The treatment setting resembles the child's natural environment as closely as possible. Because the normal "workday" for children takes place in school, the day is organized around school experiences, using these social and work interactions with peers and adults as the content for therapeutic interventions.
3. A highly consistent, interdisciplinary program is provided. To this end, a high degree of communication exists among all the staff members through direct, regularly scheduled daily meetings, through weekly chart entries, and through intramilieu memos (Zimet & Farley, 1985, p. 734).

Our day hospital treatment provides a total comprehensive treatment program that touches upon all aspects of a child's life. More specifically, its objectives are to relieve inappropriate anxiety, promote the development of adaptive skills and more realistic self-assessment, improve interpersonal relationships, increase motivation to learn, improve academic skills, and provide a safe and growth-promoting home environment for the child.

CURRENT ORGANIZATION AND FUNCTIONING

The Diagnostic Process

One full-time psychiatric social worker is in charge of the intake process (see the chapter on intake by Kayser and Tenorio). Following the intake, the child is brought in for an evaluation period of 6 weeks. A team, consisting of a child therapist, a parent or family therapist, a principal teacher, and a team leader is assigned to coordinate the evaluation process. Our standard database is obtained during this evaluation period and is fully described in a later chapter by Zimet, Farley, and Avitable. At team meetings during the evaluation process, a problem list is developed, and plans targeting each problem are developed. Necessary educational and psychological testing is obtained. An Individual Education Plan (IEP) is developed by the teacher and parents. A home visit by the team is often a part of this initial assessment (please see the chapter by Ekanger).

At the end of the 6-week evaluation period the results of the assessment and the plan for treatment are presented at a full staff meeting, plans are further refined, and a decision is made regarding treatment of the child and family. If the child continues in the program, this treatment team continues as constituted during the evaluation phase.

Team Functioning

Each child in the Day Care Center is assigned an individual therapist. This therapist meets with the child two or three times a week in developmental/cognitive/behavioral/psychodynamic child psychotherapy. We feel that by assigning an individual therapist, a message is given to the child, and that message is "We think that you are important. We are here for you. We are not *only* the agent of your parents and society." The information gained and the work done in these individual sessions is brought to the weekly team meeting. At the team meeting are the parents' therapist (or therapists), the principal teacher, and the team leader (a clinical staff member). The central activity of the team meeting is to discuss the events and activities of the previous week from each perspective (parent therapist, child therapist, classroom teacher), identify an important and salient problem, plan a course of action to help ameliorate the problem in each domain (classroom, home, child psychotherapy), and assign responsibility to team members to carry out the action. Each member comes to the team with a different perspective, and the task of the team leader is to integrate and synthesize these varied views.

Child Psychotherapy

Each child in the program is assigned an individual child psychotherapist. What happens between the therapist and child varies greatly, but usually it is some variety of psychodynamically, interpersonally oriented child psychotherapy. There is an emphasis on understanding how life experiences and important relationships influence current functioning and how major conflictual areas are acted out in present relationships. The understanding of and working through of important traumata such as loss of parents and experiences of abuse and illness are also important.

In a significant number of cases, a behavior modification contract is worked out among the therapist, the child, the parents, and other team members. The purpose of the contract and the provisions of it would likely become a focus for individual psychotherapy.

Children in our program prize their individual therapy and therapist. They often brag to other children about how good their therapist is to them.

Group Therapy with Children

Because nearly all our children have difficulty in getting along with other children, group child psychotherapy would seem important. Our efforts at group therapy have ranged from psychodynamically oriented talking groups to behaviorally oriented activities groups. Some of our more successful efforts have included group therapy around an issue that is common to a certain group of children. We have had groups that were conducted by a team consisting of a clinician and a teacher and were organized around the theme of children returning to a public school setting. We have had groups conducted by a team of two clinicians and were organized around the fact that each of the children in the group had recently lost a therapist. Each teacher and aide has some group-oriented activity during the school day, and much of this activity is oriented around the themes of consideration for others, taking another's view, taking turns, listening to others, interpersonal conflict resolution, power sharing, and self-esteem building. For more on group psychotherapy with an educational emphasis, please see the chapter on "Special Projects in the Treatment Program," by Parsons and Imhoff.

Rituals, Rules, and Regularity

When children lead chaotic lives, it is important that the treatment setting be predictable and organized. We have felt that it is necessary to mark certain events in children's lives with a public recognition. When a new child comes in, his or her teacher introduces the child to the class. He or she will already have had an introductory tour and visit. At lunchtime, there is already an assigned place to sit and eat. The child is told about lunchtime rules by the other children. All team members are assigned and in place, including the child's therapist. Often the child is welcomed into the group psychotherapy by the child letting other group members know something about him- or herself, and they, in turn, learn about the group rules and the other members. At camp, there are many campfires and awards for cooperation, making friends, helping one another, and discovering something (please see the chapter on camp by Mulligan). At the time of the child's birthday, the cook bakes a cake or pie (flavor and type of the child's choosing), and everyone sings happy birthday. At the time the child leaves the program, the teacher makes a scrapbook, complete with pictures of the child and the child's friends in the program. Written messages from staff members and children are also in the book. The child is given a gift from the Day Care Center, the teacher gives a little goodbye speech, and sometimes the child has something to say. All staff members are invited for ice cream and cake at this noontime goodbye party.

Special projects around holidays, such as Chanukah, Christmas, Easter, Presidents' Day, Martin Luther King, Jr. Day, Thanksgiving, Memorial Day, and the Fourth of July, are often organized in the classroom (please see the chapter by Parsons and Imhoff).

We always invite children to return for a visit. A high proportion of them do, often returning for lunch, and sometimes returning many years later and bringing their children and spouses with them. At the time of their return, they often have a new perspective about their current life and their previous problematic behavior and are likely to make comments such as "I can't believe what an obnoxious brat I was when I first came here. I'm surprised you people put up with me."

SUMMARY AND CONCLUSIONS

This has been the story of the birth, evolution, development, and maturing of a single day treatment program. The program today has many of the features of the original program, but significant changes are also in place. Our original intention was to answer the question, "What kinds of treatments make what kinds of differences to what kinds of children over what lengths of time, under what kinds of conditions?" Although we have only begun to approach this question in all its complexity, we have been able to describe our population, define the treatment we offer, describe some of the changes that we see, and make some conjectures about which children change the most, the least, and why. Another important feature of our program is its longevity. The program is now in its twenty-ninth year, and during this period, it has enjoyed continued support of the Division of Child Psychiatry and the Department of Psychiatry over many years and difficult times. We have also had the benefit of a highly competent and very dedicated staff and faculty, committed to the effort of providing high-quality treatment to parents and children in desperate need of our services.

REFERENCES

Ayres, A. J. (1973). *Sensory integration and learning disorders.* Los Angeles: Western Psychological Services.

Cratty, B. J. (1969). *Perceptual-motor behavior and educational processes.* Springfield, IL: Thomas.

Cratty, B. J. (1970). *Perceptual and motor development in infants and children.* New York: Macmillan.

Cruickshank, W. M. (Ed.). (1966). *The teacher of brain injured children.* Syracuse, NY: Syracuse University Press.

Cruickshank, W. M., Bentzen, F. A., Ratzeburg, F. H., & Tannhauser, M. T. (1961). *A teaching method for brain-injured and hyperactive children.* Syracuse, NY: Syracuse University Press.

Frostig, M. (1970). *Movement education: Theory and practice.* Chicago, IL: Follett Educational Corporation.

Kephart, N. C. (1964). *The slow learner in the classroom.* Columbus, OH: Charles E. Merrill.

Kirk, S. A., & Kirk, W. D. (1971). *Psycholinguistic learning disabilities: Diagnosis and remediation.* Urbana, IL: University of Illinois Press.

Zimet, S. G., & Farley, G. K. (1985). Day treatment for children in the United States. *Journal of the American Academy of Child Psychiatry, 24,* 732–738.

II

Aspects of the Clinical and Educational Programs

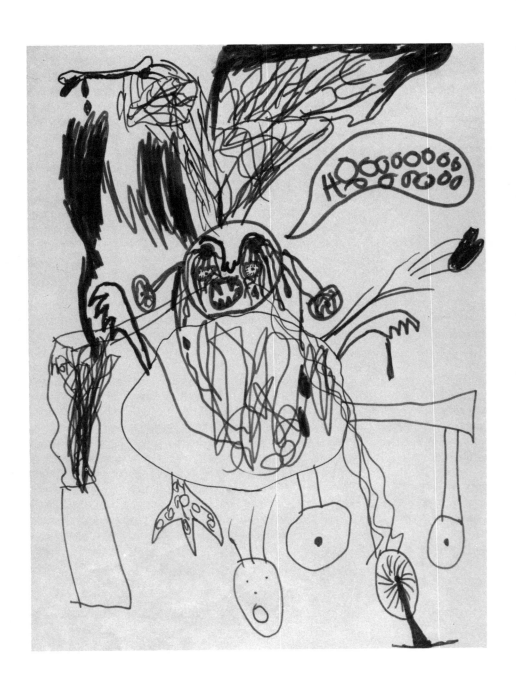

The reader will find Part II to be a rich resource of practical information and stimulating ideas. The nine chapters making up this part explore each of the issues they touch upon with a thoroughness and depth that should satisfy the reader's desire for specificity. Starting with a chapter on the intake process, "Intake as a Clinical Intervention in Day Hospital Treatment" (Chapter 2), John Kayser and Abe Tenorio do two things. First, they review the literature dealing with intake in clinical settings, and second, they describe their view of intake as a process that is integral to our treatment program. Issues regarding child advocacy and the competence of children to provide information about themselves introduce the reader to interesting areas not previously explored in this context. Both authors are psychiatric social workers who have guided the intake process at our center at separate times over the past 14 years. They bring a maturity to the subject worthy of the reader's consideration.

Charles Ekanger, assistant director and chief social worker at the Day Care Center, puts us in touch with an old and treasured assessment and treatment approach in his chapter, "Contributions of Home Visits to Patient Evaluation and Treatment" (Chapter 3). Through the use of descriptions of actual visits, we discover the clinical and personal advantages of seeing the child and family in the naturalistic setting of their home. He also examines the attitudes of the various mental health professionals toward home visits and how these attitudes influence a home visitation program. He has been at the center since its inception and, therefore, is able to provide the reader with the advantage of hindsight to this topic.

In Chapter 4, Gordon Farley describes a mainstay of our treatment program, Standby. It provides backup to staff members working directly with individuals or groups of children at times when one or more of the children loses control or isolates himself or herself and threatens the integrity of the group. The organization and implementation of this program makes up the substance of this chapter.

In "The Role of Education in Our Day Treatment Program" (Chapter 5), Sara Zimet, an educational psychologist and director of research and program evaluation at the center, and Ralph Imhoff, head teacher, provide the reader with a comprehensive description of the characteristics of the school curriculum. The assumptions underlying theory and practice are presented in the context of a program that is well integrated into all other aspects of the treatment program. The authors also discuss the concept of "parallel process," in which the relationships within the patients' families are sometimes enacted among teachers and their supervisors, teachers and their students, and among treatment team members. This chapter is rich in ideas and information.

Chapter 6 focuses on one area of the curriculum, as its title indicates: "Reading and Writing in a Therapeutic Classroom." Carol Lee invites us into her classroom and introduces us to her six students. Without pretext, she takes us through every aspect of her language program, leaving no doubt that we will recognize her, her classroom, and her students when we meet them.

Phyllis Parsons, a veteran with over 25 years of experience in teaching children with serious emotional disorders, has much to teach teachers and other mental health professionals. In her delightful chapter, "Behind the Bottom Line: A Cautionary Tale for New Teachers of Troubled and Troublesome Children" (Chapter 7), she has an uncanny way of identifying the key concerns in working with this population of children. Her wry humor does not distract from the wisdom of her advice nor from the depth of her dedication to her profession.

Sara Zimet and Geraldine Schultz, our dietitian and cook, appear to have a very good time telling us about food in the Day Treatment Program in Chapter 8. This topic is placed, first, in its broadest cultural context, and gradually we are introduced to the cast: the cook, the children, the lunchtime supervisors, the teachers, the psychotherapists, and the parents. At times we are in the kitchen; at other times we are in the cafeteria, the classroom, and the therapy room. This is a chapter that encompasses theory, research, and practice, and leaves us with a few favorite recipes as well.

"Beyond the City Limits: The Kids and Staff at Camp" (Chapter 9) describes a 1-week experience each year that appears to have important positive clinical reverberations the year around. Patricia Mulligan, one of our very talented teachers with a penchant for the out-of-doors, provides a comprehensive accounting of the planning and implementation of this program component. Beginning with a statement regarding its aims and objectives, we then move into the nuts and bolts of making this program work for the children, their families, and the center staff members. Patricia Mulligan, while addressing the routines of camp life, also discusses the concerns of the children and their families—particularly those associated with leaving home, the management of chronic medical illnesses, and the handling of embarrassing situations associated with soiling and bed-wetting. In effect, the author presents us with all that we need to know with the enthusiasm and dedication of a missionary spirit.

Over the many years our program has been operating, we have thought a great deal about why, what, and how we do what we do. Sometimes we have felt the need to change an approach, either in order to improve it or to add variety and newness to the program. We like to think of ourselves as solving problems creatively and rationally. In Chapter 10, we bring Part II to a close with "Special Projects in the Treatment Program: Their Birth, Development, and Occasional Demise." Phyllis Parsons and Ralph Imhoff review six of these projects in careful detail. They may motivate the reader to do something similar or caution the reader away; that decision is left in your hands.

2

Intake as a Clinical Intervention in Day Hospital Treatment

JOHN A. KAYSER and ABE E. TENORIO

INTRODUCTION

The increasing volume and complexity of referrals made to the Day Care Center in recent years has necessitated a careful examination of the role of intake in our program. Each year we receive between 60 and 100 referrals, which far exceeds the program's capacity of 23 children. These referrals come from a wide range of sources, including public and private schools, social service departments, juvenile courts, outpatient clinics, community mental health centers, inpatient psychiatric hospitals, residential treatment centers, other day treatment programs, pediatric health services, as well as from other clinical units at the University of Colorado Health Sciences Center. Often many agencies and service providers are involved with a given family. Each agency may have a different perspective regarding the need for day treatment, and this may or may not be shared by the family being referred. Thus each referral presents unique features, not only in terms of the problems presented by the child and the family, but also in terms of the helping systems that already may be providing services.

JOHN A. KAYSER • Graduate School of Social Work, University of Denver, Denver, Colorado 80208. **ABE E. TENORIO** • The Day Care Center, Department of Psychiatry, University of Colorado Health Sciences Center, Denver, Colorado 80262.

Many challenges are encountered in the intake process in determining which referrals are clinically appropriate for day treatment and which are realistic for our program to accept. For example, many families, whose children potentially are appropriate for day treatment, come to the intake interview with negative or mistrustful attitudes toward mental health. These attitudes may be based on several factors: (a) the child or family's previous unsuccessful treatment; (b) the parents' dissatisfaction with the helping professionals or agencies already involved; (c) the child or family's misconceptions about mental health or illness; (d) cultural differences in attitudes toward mental health treatment; and (e) the parents' fears about removing their child from the local school and community.

One challenge is to engage families at intake in determining whether day treatment can be helpful, given their previous ideas and experiences regarding mental health interventions. Other challenges faced also may include securing the financial and other practical resources necessary to admit a child for day hospital treatment.

In the pages that follow, we have attempted to describe a variety of approaches in meeting these intake challenges. Some of these approaches are generic in nature and could be applied to most child clinical settings (e.g., outpatient and partial hospitalization); several are based on the experience of other treatment settings; and one is based on the Day Care Center's experience of intake as it has developed during the past 27 years. In the last section, case material will be presented to illustrate the problems we have encountered and the types of clinical interventions we have provided during the intake process.

FEATURES OF INTAKE INTERVIEWS

The child mental health literature has focused on the intake process predominantly in terms of outpatient treatment or in terms of the activities of individual practitioners. According to Staver and LaForge (1975), most of the literature on intake with children has come from adult psychiatry and social services rather than from child psychiatry, possibly because "child patients do not usually refer themselves, complain about waiting lists, or demand equal treatment or a voice in intake decisions" (p. 592). In addition, a traditional view held in child psychiatry has been that disturbed children are not reliable informants about their problems (Werkman, 1965). This also may contribute to the lack of attention given in the literature to intake procedures with children.

Intake, as used in the child outpatient mental health literature, usually refers to an interview that encompasses one or more of the following four functions: (a) giving and getting information, (b) reviewing and determining suitability for admission, (c) carrying out a comprehensive evaluation, and (d) preparing and planning for treatment. In the paragraphs that follow, each of these functions is discussed separately. In addition, the interrelationships among the separate intake functions are discussed in terms of a sequence of progressive stages whereby children and their families gain access to day hospital services.

The Functions of Intake

The Information Interview. Typically, the first contact with a treatment program is requests for information from inquiring families, professionals, and/or agencies. The purpose of the information interview, which often is done over the telephone, is *to provide preliminary information about the program and obtain initial information about the child and family.* For example, general information on institutional policies, the population served, availability of openings, the scope of treatment services, and goals of the program is commonly shared. If the inquiry is regarding a specific child, a synopsis of the problem and family situation is obtained. Typically, these interviews are brief and do not involve an ongoing or continuous relationship between the intake staff and individuals inquiring about help.

The Application Interview. The application interview typically is the first face-to-face contact between a treatment program and the referred family and child. The overall purpose is *to review requests for help and to make a preliminary determination as to whether a referred family is eligible for services* (Gill, Newman, & Sommers, 1954). In addition, the application interview reviews with prospective users the feasibility of providing treatment services. Usually this means identifying practical and financial resources that are needed and available to make the delivery of services possible (e.g., third-party payment and transportation), and determining the extent and kind of assistance referred families require in obtaining these resources. The application interview, which also is brief, lays the foundation for the clinical services (e.g., evaluation and treatment) that may be provided at some later date (Staver & LaForge, 1975).

The Evaluation Interview. The evaluation interview occurs when the primary purpose of intake is *to make a psychiatric assessment of the referred child and family.* It is likely to involve one or more diagnostic interviews with both child and parents over an extended period of time and may be regarded as the beginning of a facility's formal clinical services. The evaluation focuses on answering specific diagnostic question, such as:

Does the referred child present any disorder or abnormality of emotion, behavior, or relationship? If so, what is the nature and extent of this disorder (Rutter & Graham, 1968)? Is the child's or family's disorder one that the treatment facility is equipped to handle (Coleman, Short, & Hirschberg, 1948)? In other words, the evaluation interview is meant to provide a comprehensive initial understanding of the problem requiring professional intervention and to suggest effective interventions for needed change (Berliner, 1977). This interview, therefore, is likely to be the beginning development of a helping relationship with prospective clients (Gill *et al.*, 1954).

The Pretreatment Interview. The pretreatment interview takes place when the primary purpose of the initial contact is *to prepare children and parents for treatment* (Blanchard, 1940). This interview typically extends over one or more sessions, with the specific focus on establishing an ongoing therapeutic relationship with the patient (Coleman *et al.*, 1948).

The impetus to seek professional help often stems from family crises, either with individual family members or with the collective family unit. Pretreatment interviews are likely to center on helping family members deal with feelings of helplessness, anxiety, or guilt that may arise around feelings about the need for professional help and/or the form of needed treatment (Coleman *et al.*, 1948). The patients are encouraged, therefore, to express their fantasies or preconceived ideas about therapy and/or the treatment facility. This information also contributes to an assessment of the defenses and resistances an individual or family group may bring to the therapeutic process (e.g., the extent to which denial or rationalization about the presence of problems exist), which helps in the anticipation of the course of treatment and in deciding on recommendations for specific interventions (Coleman *et al.*, 1948).

Stages of the Intake Process

As can be seen, the individual intake functions have been regarded in the child mental health literature as separate and independent of each other. However, it is probably more useful to regard these functions as progressive stages in the intake process, the goal of which is admission. Ideally, sharing information about a treatment program should lead to families making application for services. This, in turn, should lead to evaluation and preparation of families and children for treatment. In reality, this sequence is not always followed. However, conceptualizing the intake process in this fashion allows practitioners to focus their clinical interventions on helping referred families negotiate the extent of their involvement with a treatment setting at each stage of the intake process. For example, some families will conclude their involvement after the information interview, having determined that day treatment services are not what they need. Other families will progress onward making application for service.

Based on the evaluation interview, some families will end their involvement because day treatment services have been determined not to be appropriate for the child. Other families will move from the evaluation interview to the pretreatment interview, in which final preparations and decisions are made about undertaking day treatment. We now turn to an examination of how the various functions of intake have been incorporated into different models of intake used in children's day treatment centers.

SOME MODELS OF INTAKE AS DESCRIBED IN THE LITERATURE

Although day hospital care for children has been with us since the 1940s (Zimet & Farley, 1985), little attention has been given to the intake process in the literature describing these programs. In the past 10 years, for example, one paper was found that describes an intake model in the United States (Tovey & Morton, 1985), and three others were found that describe models in Western Europe (Arajarvi & Oranen, 1983; Zimet, 1987, 1988). Each of these models is summarized later along with a more detailed description of the procedures used at our day treatment center. Each model approaches the intake process as an extension of their total treatment program and provides an example of intake as a clinical intervention. In those countries outside the United States, intake into day treatment usually is preceded by intake into the mental health system, where referral to a specific service follows. In most countries the referral begins with the least restrictive setting considered first. Thus by the time a family reaches a day treatment unit, the likelihood is that they have already been through some of the steps of at least one other intake procedure.

A Multiple-Impact Model

Tovey and Morton (1985) have developed an intake evaluation process in a day treatment program for children 3 to 12 years old, based on the family systems model of "multiple-impact therapy" (MacGregor, 1962). The entire family or household of the referred child meets with a team of therapists for 5 or more hours on a single day. The family is seen both as a total group as well as individually. The objectives of this all-day process are to develop a "family plan" with the family members participating actively in describing their current level of functioning and in formulating what they want to get out of the treatment program. At the end of the daylong evaluation, team members share their observations and recommendations with the family. The family is encouraged to respond to what they have heard by asking for clarification and by expressing areas of agreement and disagreement. If the family agrees to proceed with treatment, a limited number of goals is set so that the family and the team are not left feeling overwhelmed. Concomitant to developing this plan, an alliance is being established that provides the basis for the therapeutic work ahead (Tovey & Morton, 1985).

An Intensified Contact Therapy Model

Arajarvi and Oranen (1983) describe an intake approach in a day psychiatric unit for children 9 to 14 years old in Helsinki, Finland. This initial engagement with the child and his or her family is referred to as "intensified contact therapy." This procedure extends over several weeks and has, as its primary goal, the preparation of the entire family for day hospital treatment. The purpose of the first family meeting is to assess the family's motivation for treatment and goals for treatment. This is done through an exchange of information, at which time the family describes the situation that brought them to the day unit, and, in turn, the family is told about the day unit. If the family expresses continuing interest in day treatment, a visit to the day unit is arranged. Additional meetings also are scheduled in order to explore issues related to family members' fears, fantasies, and ambivalence about treatment and to answer any questions about the treatment process. The exploration of the conflictual feelings held by each family member is given particular emphasis.

Prior to the final phase of the intake process, a home visit is made in order to observe the child's living situation and the interactions among all of the family members. These visits have helped the day unit staff adjust their perceptions of family relationships gained in the unfamiliar setting of the day unit.

The final phase of this model of intake is a discussion with the family, at which time the family decides on whether or not to enter the day treatment program.

Other European Models

Zimet (1987, 1988) studied day psychiatric treatment for emotionally handicapped children in six Western European countries: England, France, The Netherlands, Norway, Sweden, and Switzerland. Although many differences may exist with and among these countries in their day hospital intake procedures, the following list summarizes their common elements:

1. Intake procedures tend to be spread over time, ranging from 6 weeks to 6 months.
2. The evaluation process is likely to focus on the entire family unit as well as on the identified child patient.
3. The evaluation of the child is extensive and thorough, using structured play interviews, psychological, academic, and language tests, measures of perceptual–sensorimotor skills, and observations in the child's home and community school as well as in the day unit.
4. In some countries, several families are evaluated at the same time. This permits observations of peer interactions and interactions with various staff members.
5. Typically, parents are required to give a verbal commitment to participate in the extended evaluation or sign a written contract that stipulates the requirements of their participation in the treatment program.

THE INTAKE MODEL AT THE DAY CARE CENTER

Our View of the Intake Process

Our program sees intake as a broad service, encompassing all of the four intake functions described earlier, and each involving clinical interventions. For example, in the information interview, families are helped to obtain any of the resources they may need for admission to the program. By intervening in this way, we are demonstrating our concern for their well-being, a first step toward building trust. Additional examples of clinical interventions are given later. We believe that by establishing a strong alliance with the family during the intake process, we may be able to prevent an early withdrawal from treatment.

Clinical interventions also occur with families who, we believe, are not appropriate for our treatment program. In these instances, we provide the family with assistance in finding a more appropriate treatment setting in the community.

During the application interview, clinical interventions are likely to occur where we simply listen attentively to families who are in distress, when we help them clarify the type of service they want, and when we assist them in deciding whether our program is appropriate for them. They also occur when we respond sensitively to their anxieties about seeking day treatment (Staver & LaForge, 1975) and help them determine if they can afford it.

In the pretreatment interview, a working alliance between referred families and our program develops. This alliance serves not only as the foundation for joint decision making about admission into the program but provides a therapeutic framework within which the family can gradually reveal its conflicts and difficulties. Thus this gradual development of the therapeutic relationship helps prevent the family from disclosing its problems prematurely (Solomon, 1977).

Our Administrative Structure

Our day treatment program is one of several mental health services provided by the Department of Psychiatry at the University of Colorado's Health Sciences Center campus. We treat 5- to 12-year-old children and their families with moderate to severe emotional and behavioral disorders, who reside in the Greater Denver metropolitan area. We believe that effective clinical interventions during the intake process require both a coherent intake policy as well as a clearly defined authority for decision making assigned to the intake director (Staver & LaForge, 1975). Our intake policy is formulated by the Intake Committee composed of the Day Care Center's director (a child psychiatrist), the head teacher (an educator), and the director of intake services (a senior clinical social worker). The committee meets once a week. It delegates the following responsibilities to the intake director: (a) screening initial applicants and accepting those who will continue through our intake process; (b) making recommendations to the intake committee regarding the child's date of admission, the selection of personnel for treatment teams, and the child's educational placement in the program; (c) supervising the social work interns assigned to work with new referrals; (d) developing referral sources; and (e) clarifying the nature and scope of our treatment program to parents and families seeking help as well as to referring agencies and professionals.

The Chronology of Our Intake Process

1. The intake director obtains the initial information about a patient and his or her family over the telephone. If the referral is appropri-

ate but there is no opening, the child's name is placed on our waiting list. An important function of the intake director is to maintain contact with the families. When an opening occurs, a more complete intake interview with the child and family is scheduled. During this interview, information related to the child and family's problems and areas of strength is gathered.

2. In the meetings that follow, the intake committee reviews new information gathered on each of the referrals and the recommendations made by the intake director regarding their disposition. Decisions are made regarding their status, whether they will move to the next stage of the intake process or be referred elsewhere. The status of existing referrals is monitored at these meetings as well.

3. When a child and his or her family are accepted for further evaluation, the parents are asked to complete all the forms in our intake packet. This packet contains various authorizations and release-of-information forms that are needed to obtain pertinent records for the child's clinical chart from other agencies and/or professionals who may be involved. The packet also contains a developmental history questionnaire, a child behavior checklist (Achenbach & Edelbrock, 1983), and a parent symptom checklist (Derogatis, 1983), all of which are collected as part of the Day Care Center's standard database (see chapter by Zimet, Farley, and Avitable). If needed, the intake director may help parents to complete these materials.

4. In order to prepare our staff members for the child's trial placement in the program, the intake director prepares a written summary of presenting problems for discussion at our next weekly staff meeting. At the same time, the intake director assembles a multidisciplinary team to conduct the evaluation. The team consists of (a) the team leader (either a staff social worker or child psychiatrist); (b) an educator (the child's teacher); and (c) two clinicians, the child's therapist and the parents' and/or family's therapist. This same group of people will continue to function as the treatment team should the child be accepted into our program.

5. Meanwhile, the finance committee, consisting of our intake director, the assistant director, and the administrative officer, meets with the child's parents. They discuss the cost of treatment and explore the various avenues available for meeting this cost. In most cases, parents are not familiar either with the mental health benefits provided by their insurance carrier or with other sources of support such as (a) Medicaid, (b) Supplemental Security Income, (c) contract purchases of day treatment by local school districts or social services departments, or (d) partial support from a subsidized adoption agreement. To obtain any consideration of these alternatives and in order to establish their out-of-pocket fees, parents must provide us with complete documentation of their in-

come. With this information at hand, the finance committee does everything in its power to help a family obtain support to meet their financial obligations to us.

6. The comprehensive evaluation involves collecting information on the child's functioning at home, in his or her school, in individual psychotherapy, and in the day hospital milieu. Parents and other family members are interviewed at the center, and a home visit may be made. The trial placement extends over 2 to 3 weeks and ends with a staff review conference, where a decision is made as to whether to accept the child and family or to refer them elsewhere. This meeting is followed by an interpretive hour with the parents, where the family situation and treatment plan are discussed. If the child and family are seen as being helped by our program, they arrive at a joint decision regarding the child's continuation in the program.

Clinical Interventions during Intake

Case material from the Day Care Center's referrals has been selected to illustrate typical clinical interventions that are likely to occur in the intake process.

During the Information Interview. Many families are unfamiliar with mental health services. When information requests are received, the intake director helps families to understand the range of services available, both within our institution as well as in the community-at-large. In effect, parents are helped to make an informed decision about which level of care to explore. As the following vignette shows, ascertaining the nature of the request for help is a crucial task at the information stage of intake.

> A long-distance phone call was received from a parent in Texas inquiring about the admission of her child into the program. As the Intake Director described the program, it became clear that the mother already had decided to pursue residential care for her child, and was not open to exploring day hospitalization. The mother was assisted in making contact with a county department of social services to obtain further information about residential facilities in Colorado.

During the Application Interview

Financial Arrangements. As stated earlier, clinical interventions made as part of fulfilling the application function differ according to whether the referral is appropriate or not appropriate for our program. For appropriate referrals, clinical interventions often focus on securing the practical resources required for a child's admission. This type of intervention enables day treatment not only to begin but to be sustained. The following case example focuses on one of the concerns that many families face, that of securing adequate financial resources.

> A 5-year-old boy had been accepted for evaluation. Although the family had 100% insurance coverage for day hospital treatment, it was discovered during intake that the life-time maximum insurance benefit would be exhausted after only a brief treatment period. To avoid interrupting treatment, the intake director helped the parents apply for the Supplemental Security Income (SSI) program, which provided Medicaid coverage for the child's psychiatric treatment.

Transportation Arrangements. Another problem faced by many families is providing for the daily transportation to and from the center. In some cases, this is due to conflicting work and Day Care Center schedules. In other cases, either parents cannot afford a car, or public transportation is not available. As the following vignette demonstrates, sometimes more than one transportation resource has to be tapped.

> A 5-year-old girl had no apparent means of transportation to the center because of her parents' work schedule and the distance between their home and the center (about 25 miles). The intake director, therefore, negotiated with two agencies: (a) the Red Cross in the family's home county to provide a morning ride to the center 4 days a week; and (b) a transportation service paid for by the county social services agency, for the after-school transportation of the child to the mother's place of employment 4 days a week. For the 1 remaining day left, her parents were able to make other arrangements for getting her to and from the center.

Referral Elsewhere. Not accepting a referral presents us with a special form of clinical intervention. As noted earlier, an initial determination is made regarding whether the child's presenting problems fall within the program's treatment capabilities. Children with severe autistic features, severe mental retardation, gross developmental delays, lack of speech, out-of-control behavior requiring daily seclusion and/or constant physical restraint, or those with severe and acute medical problems generally are not considered appropriate for our day hospital. As the following case example illustrates, clarifying the limits of our treatment program and responding sensitively to parents' feelings of disappointment when a referral is not accepted may be the first step in the parents' recognition of the extent and severity of the child's problems.

An autistic 11-year-old boy had been successfully placed for 5 years in his school district's program for autistic children. He moved outside the district and was placed in a program that was not capable of providing him with the care that he needed. As a result, he had become totally unmanageable both at school and at home. Thus he was referred to us by this therapist. In addition to the fact that the school district did not have a class for children with his disorder and that the boy may have been upset by his dual moves from familiar to unfamiliar settings (home and school), there was the additional concern that his condition was deteriorating and that he might have to be placed in residential care. His mother feared this latter possibility and was prepared to fight it. The problem, as we saw it, was that given an appropriate setting in his neighborhood community, he would be able to function as well as he had done before and would not require the "more restrictive" environment of the day care center or of a residential placement. Intake interventions focused on helping the mother consider not only the child's immediate situation but also his long-term education and psychological needs. Therefore, we recommended that mother and therapist work with the current school program to develop an effective treatment plan for the boy. Some months later, we learned that they had followed our recommendations, the school district had created a program for children with autism, and the child's behavior and overall functioning had improved markedly.

During the Comprehensive Evaluation. Clinical interventions during the evaluation function occur (a) when the level of treatment needed for effective intervention as assessed by our staff differs from the level of treatment the family desires; (b) when there are unresolved questions regarding the family's ability to follow through with the treatment program's expectations; and (c) when the degree of immediate risk to the child and/or the family is higher than the program can manage.

Level of Care. Day hospitalization is seen as one of several treatment modalities available on a continuum of mental health services for children and their families. A common assessment made at intake, therefore, is whether the presenting problems can be treated in a more or less restrictive setting than day treatment, such as in an inpatient or residential setting, or as an outpatient. Thus our intake director makes a preliminary assessment as to whether the presenting problems require the level of care provided by day treatment. However, the type of help the family is seeking may differ from the type of help the clinical setting we are recommending (Lazare, Eisenthal, & Wasserman, 1975), as the following vignette illustrates.

A self-referred family contacted the program regarding their 6-year-old daughter who had had numerous and unsuccessful trials of outpatient psychotherapy. The parents presented their situation with a desperate urgency, demanding the child's immediate admission into the program. At the same time, however, the parents became argumentative about the evaluation procedures and level of care offered by the program. Specifically, the parents emphatically refused to participate in parent or family assessment interviews, insisting that the child—not they—should be the focus of the problem. The parents' unwillingness to negotiate a compromise precluded admission to our program.

Meeting the Program's Expectations. The ability of the family to follow through on the expectations of our treatment program also is assessed during the intake evaluation. The intake director reviews the past history of treatment and the family's ability to follow previous treatment recommendations. As the following vignette illustrates, considerable diagnostic information on the family's overall functioning can be learned from observing how they comply with required intake steps.

A 5-year-old boy was referred by a social services caseworker. Although the maternal grandmother was the primary caretaker since the child's birth, the biological mother retained legal custody. At first, we felt that it would be appropriate for the mother to meet with us regularly. However, the mother's ambivalent relationship and erratic contact with the child posed significant barriers to treatment. In addition, mother repeatedly failed to show up at our scheduled intake interviews. Thus a plan was negotiated with social services to involve the maternal grandmother in the therapeutic contacts with our center.

Assessing Risk. Assessing the degree of immediate risk presented by a child and/or family often means that the intake director functions in the role of a crisis worker. Because the average length of time between referral and admission ranges from 3 to 6 months, the intake director must determine whether a family realistically can cope with a waiting period or whether immediate treatment is required. In the following vignette, a family contacted us in a state of extreme distress involving an incident of child abuse.

A 30-year-old single mother who had recently moved to Denver contacted us for help with her youngest child, a 7-year-old hyperactive boy. Following the first contact, mother called the intake director again in a state of extreme distress. She stated that she had just "beat" her son because he had let the family dog out of their fenced yard and the dog had run away. The mother and son were given a same-day appointment, during which time the mother's abuse of the child was evident. Mother described having sat on her son's chest, repeatedly slapping his face and screaming in rage. The child's cheeks were bright red with finger imprints easily identifiable.

The mother cried and expressed deep remorse over her actions. The intake director explained that the first step in gaining assistance was reporting the child abuse to the proper social services department, as required by Colorado statute. After much support, the mother called The Denver Department of Social Services from the intake director's office. The next step involved short- and long-term planning. For the short term, mother and son were referred to our outpatient clinic so that therapy could begin immediately. For the long term, the child was placed on our waiting list for admission as soon as an opening occurred.

During the Pretreatment Stage. Frequently, referrals contain treatment barriers that must be addressed if day treatment is to succeed. As Kaplan (1952) observes, referrals for child treatment may occur as a result of an unrecognized impasse between families and the agencies and/or professionals involved with them. Identifying and removing these obstacles is an integral part of the intake treatment process and enhances a family's readiness to enter day treatment. In the following example, the intake director was the catalyst in helping a family and agency identify and resolve an unrecognized stumbling block to day treatment.

An adopted 10-year-old girl who was hospitalized for 1 year in a private psychiatric hospital was referred to the program for continued treatment. Her parents were in the process of getting a divorce. They were bitter, antagonistic, and unable to communicate directly with each other. A dispute over their daughter's custody posed a major obstacle to the progress of future treatment. During intake, it became obvious that each parent used the daughter to antagonize the other. Their differences over her care included how she should be disciplined and what food she should be allowed to eat. The intake committee took the position that the child would not be accepted for further evaluation until there was a resolution regarding her custody. Over the course of 2 months, the intake director worked with the parents, their attorneys, and the hospital staff to achieve an agreement that granted temporary custody to the father and regular visitation with the mother. This preadmission work served not only as the basis for the permanent custody orders but also enabled the child to make a smooth transition from inpatient care to day hospital treatment.

CONCLUSION

The scope of intake functions can be defined narrowly or broadly. The Day Care Center has defined intake as involving many functions. It attempts to integrate clinical assessment and treatment functions with the information gathering and applications functions. In conclusion, intake procedures are probably characteristic of the setting in which they are carried out. They are likely to reflect the purpose or mission of the treatment facility, its administrative structure, its treatment orientation, as well as the sources of available funding.

REFERENCES

Achenbach, T. M., & Edelbrock, C. (1983). *Manual for the Child Behavior Checklist and revised Child Behavior Profile.* Burlington: University of Vermont.

Arajarvi, T., & Oranen, A. M. (1983). First contacts with a family whose child is to be admitted to the child psychiatry day ward. *Acta Paedo-psychiatrica, 49,* 119–126.

Berliner, A. K. (1977). Fundamentals of intake interviewing. *Child Welfare, 56,* 665–675.

Blanchard, P. (1940). The importance of the first interviews in therapeutic work with children. *Smith College Studies in Social Work, 10,* 277–284.

Coleman, J. V., Short, G. B., & Hirschberg, J. C. (1948). The intake interview as the beginning of psychiatric treatment in children's cases. *American Journal of Psychiatry, 105,* 183–186.

Derogatis, L. R. (1983). *SCL-90-R: Administration, scoring and procedures manual.* Towson, MD: Clinical Psychometric Research.

Gill, M., Newman, R., & Sommers, M. (1954). *The initial interview in psychiatric practice.* New York: International Universities Press.

Kaplan, M. (1952). Problems between a referring source and a child psychiatry clinic. *The Quarterly Journal of Child Behavior, 4,* 80–96.

Lazare, A., Eisenthal, S., & Wasserman, L. (1975). The customer approach to patienthood. *Archives of General Psychiatry, 32,* 553–558.

MacGregor, R. (1962). Multiple impact psychotherapy with families. *Family Process, 1,* 15–29.

Rutter, M., & Graham, P. (1968). The reliability and validity of the psychiatric assessment of the child I: Interview with the child. *British Journal of Psychiatry, 114,* 563–579.

Solomon, M. A. (1977). The staging of family treatment: An approach to developing the therapeutic alliance. *Journal of Marriage and Family Counseling, 3,* 59–66.

Staver, N., & LaForge, E. (1975). Intake as a conflict area in clinic function. *Journal of the American Academy of Child Psychiatry, 14,* 689–599.

Tovey, R., & Morton, J. (1985). Adapting multiple impact therapy for day treatment intake. *Child Welfare, 64,* 421–426.

Werkman, S. L. (1965). The psychiatric diagnostic interview with children. *American Journal of Orthopsychiatry, 35,* 764–771.

Zimet, S. G. (1987). *Day psychiatric treatment for emotionally handicapped children, Part I: Norway, Sweden, and The Netherlands.* Unpublished report. The World Rehabilitation Fund, Inc., 400 East 34th Street, New York, New York.

Zimet, S. G. (1988). *Day psychiatric treatment for emotionally handicapped children, Part II: England, Switzerland, and France.* Unpublished report. The World Rehabilitation Fund, Inc., 400 East 34th Street, New York, New York.

Zimet, S. G., & Farley, G. K. (1985). Day treatment for children in the United States: An overview. *Journal of the American Academy of Child Psychiatry, 24,* 732–738.

3

Contributions of Home Visits to Patient Evaluation and Treatment

CHARLES A. EKANGER

INTRODUCTION

The contributions from home visits has long been recognized at the Day Care Center as a significant and meaningful adjunct to traditional evaluation and treatment procedures. Prior to the introduction of home visits, a child's initial evaluation at the Day Care Center primarily involved the assessment of identified emotional and adjustment problems through standard medical, psychological, and educational testing procedures as well as psychiatric interviews and review of referral information. In the process of accumulating and interpreting data from these sources, it was quite natural to consider questions related to organicity, nurturance patterns, and family history. However important these factors were in a child's psychosocial evaluation, there was the ever-present risk that they be viewed apart from the context of the patient's daily life environment.

The ideas for this chapter originally appeared in a paper by the author and Georgia Westervelt in 1967 entitled, "Contributions of Observations in Naturalistic Settings to Clinical and Educational Practice." It was published in the *Journal of Special Education, 1*, pp. 207–218.

CHARLES A. EKANGER • The Day Care Center, Department of Psychiatry, University of Colorado Health Sciences Center, Denver, Colorado 80262.

Within several years of the initial opening of the Day Care Center as a day hospital program, an attempt was made to develop a broader understanding of each child's home environment through systematic visits to the homes of all patients being evaluated for possible treatment. Existing services included psychotherapy and academic programming for all child patients, as well as office visits with parents and other family members.

Six of the initial 14 families who received home visits had co-therapists assigned to the family. Among these co-therapists were the program director, a staff psychiatrist, a psychiatric resident, and three psychiatric nurses. Each made a home visit with a staff social worker. The other eight home visits were made individually by social work staff members. For some participants, these visits represented an unaccustomed approach to the assessment process; for other staff members home visits had been a familiar procedure in previous work settings. Generally, those without prior home visiting experience initially tended to express anxiety about contacting families in their homes and expected to be viewed as intruders or detectives. Much of the expressed apprehension appeared to stem from therapists' own personal discomfort in seeing patients in a context other than the familiar office setting.

The proposed home visits were, in fact, well received by the families involved. Parents and children both appeared to understand that the visits reflected a genuine interest in getting to know, understand, and support them more fully. After several families had been visited, other children in the program began asking when someone could come to visit their home. As systematic visits were initiated, these contacts were expected to (a) test the family's motivation for treatment; (b) illustrate the child's everyday reality; (c) demonstrate typical family interactions, discipline, and limit setting; (d) clarify our impressions of the family environment; (e) provide us with supplementary information; and (f) strengthen the impact of treatment on the child patients and their families. In some instances, all of these outcomes were accomplished; in others, only a few. For illustrative purposes, however, only a few of those listed above are discussed next.

THE CLARIFICATION OF OUR IMPRESSIONS

The following descriptions illustrate how impressions and observations were clarified through direct contact with the patients' home and community environment in a way that could not have been duplicated through office interviewing.

At the time of intake, Dick lived with his parents and a younger brother in a geographically isolated government housing project. Their home was a modest, well-maintained two-bedroom frame house. It was nestled within a cluster of 16 houses in a mountain valley surrounded by a sheer wall of rock to one side and rugged hills and trees to the other. All of the houses extended on either side of a single street that had only one entrance from a winding gravel road off a main highway. This cluster of homes was located only a short distance from a power plant where all of the men in the housing project were employed. There were no stores nearby, making it necessary to travel 15 miles to purchase even a loaf of bread. Furnishings were limited primarily to basic items, attractively arranged to make for a comfortable, homey atmosphere. One of the father's hobbies, collecting guns, was easily confirmed by the gunrack on the livingroom wall. When commenting on the vast expanse of open country surrounding the houses, we were told that Dick spent much of his time roaming about and exploring the area by himself. One of Dick's special interests was building tree houses. It became a special point of interest during our guided tour of the premises by Dick to see one of the houses he had built extending daringly over the edge of a steep cliff.

As you can see, visiting Dick's home added significant data and impressions related to the physical and psychological climate that he experienced on a daily basis. These data had both immediate and continuing impact on both individual and family therapy sessions. For example, early in family treatment, it became apparent that the tree house built on the edge of the cliff reflected Dick's identification with his father's need for presenting outward appearances of strength, daring, and bravery. In addition, Dick's father reacted to any expression of feelings as an expression of weakness. Thus two of the goals in therapy for Dick and his family were to secure Dick's safety and to enable Dick and his father to experience a wider range of self-expression.

The observations made on a visit to Vance's home stood in sharp contrast with those made of Dick's family. This visit occurred during Vance's intake evaluation. It clearly dramatized the extent to which certain attitudes and behavior had come to permeate this family's way of life.

In spite of an adequate middle-class income, Vance's family had allowed their home to deteriorate to the point of looking like a ghost house. The weather-beaten exterior left no evidence of housepaint, whereas interior walls had large unrepaired holes in the plaster. The furniture within the home was very beaten and worn. There was no visible evidence of family pride in the appearance of their home. A huge, well-trained watchdog was kept at bay during our visit. We were told that the dog provided them with protection from window peekers and unwelcome visitors.

Against the background of other referral information, these observations drove home the reality of this family's propensity for controversial, nonconformist, eyebrow-raising conduct in their community. The watchdog also provided a superb example of the defensiveness, suspicion, and paranoid thinking that prevailed in this family's perception of the outside world. We understood more clearly the relationship between this family's place in their community and the defiant, negative behavior exhibited by Vance at our center.

PROVIDING US WITH SUPPLEMENTARY INFORMATION

The impressions secured through home visits complemented, clarified, and sometimes revised pictures previously obtained through more traditional office contacts (Norris-Shortle & Cohen, 1987; Woods, 1988). This is illustrated through a description of Paul's family.

> Paul, a rather effeminate 10-year-old boy, was initially referred to the Day Care Center with a severe school phobia. Up to the time of our home visit, little information had been collected about the interactional patterns of his family. During our visit, we noted that he shared a bedroom with his two older sisters, and unlike them, he did not have age-appropriate toys and equipment to play with. We also noted from seeing him interact with his parents and sisters that he was treated as the family baby and not allowed to do things on his own or to express preferences.

As a result of observing Paul's passive and nonexpressive interactions with his family, specific changes resulted in psychotherapy with Paul and his parents. Deliberate focus was placed on the significant differences that existed in role expectations of Paul at home and at the center. Paul responded with consciousness of his own ambivalent feelings about growing up and began gradually to agitate for changes on his own behalf. Several months later, he was sleeping in a room of his own and was riding a newly acquired bicycle to and from the center without continuing to depend on his mother for transportation. In effect, the home visit not only provided additional observational data but also mobilized changes in programming on a very practical level (Norris-Shortle & Cohen, 1987; Woods, 1988).

REEVALUATING OUR CLINICAL IMPRESSIONS

It was anticipated that existing clinical impressions would be supported or revised through home visits. This happened in Paul's case, as described. It also came about with Karen, who was 8 years old. A visit to Karen's foster home demonstrated how discrepancies and inconsistencies may occur between the reporting of behavior or circumstances in interviews and impressions received from direct observation.

Through office interviews, Karen's therapist had heard numerous descriptions of family interactions that suggested closeness and considerable sharing of time and activities. In visiting her foster home, however, the therapist was surprised to discover that Karen's bedroom, where she spent several hours alone each day in isolated play or TV viewing, was located in the basement. This arrangement, though adequate from a physical standpoint, effected marked physical isolation and separation from her foster parents.

The observations made in visiting Karen's home opened the door for discussions about family relationships that continued in subsequent appointments. The foster parents explained that this had been Karen's own choice of rooms when she came to live with them because she wanted to share it with another foster child already in the home. When encouraged to consider the implications of this isolation for Karen, now that she was the only child living there, her foster mother asked Karen if she would like to move into a vacant bedroom on the first floor. Before long, however, it became apparent that her foster mother was not able to recognize her own feelings of rejection that led to giving Karen double messages. Further substantiation of this was later provided when Karen related how the choice of moving upstairs would have meant leaving behind her toys and television privileges. Karen's response to these conditions was to remain in the basement. Both Karen and her foster mother rationalized that the final choice had been Karen's, and in this way they avoided having to deal with their underlying feelings of rejection and guilt.

BROADENING OUR UNDERSTANDING OF THE CHILD'S EVERYDAY REALITY

The home visits had the effect of broadening our understanding of each child's life outside the clinical setting of our center. In the overall program, this served to offer a perspective in thinking about individual children and promoted a greater appreciation for the "whole person" in a larger environment. The visit to Sheldon's home is one example of this outcome.

> Sheldon, a 7-year-old black child, lived with his parents in a two-bedroom brick home with a neatly trimmed lawn in both the front- and backyard. As they showed us around the house, Sheldon's parents proudly announced that they had finally realized their dream of leaving a public housing project and moving into this house, their own home, situated in an attractive neighborhood with families of their own racial and ethnic background. They said that they were especially pleased that their son could be raised in a safe and caring neighborhood, in contrast to the one they had left behind.

In the course of the daily interchange between our staff and our child patients, it was easy to overlook the significant differences that existed for some children between their home environment and the environment of our center. In the preceding example, the home visit was a reminder of the existence of the subsystems (Spiegel & Bell, 1959) that Sheldon experienced beyond our center and about which we knew very little. Through this contact, our primarily white staff also became more conscious of the possible implications for Sheldon of moving each day between a predominantly black and a predominantly white community. This visit also provided a new awareness into feelings held by Sheldon's parents about the neighborhood in which they were now living, in contrast to the one from which they had recently moved.

STRENGTHENING THE TREATMENT PROGRAM

It was anticipated that home visits would strengthen ongoing therapeutic efforts, develop a closer working relationship between families and the staff of the center, and lead to possible changes in educational and clinical approaches, both to child patients and their families (Norris-Shortle & Cohen, 1987; Woods, 1988). The case of 6-year-old Wanda illustrates each of these points.

> Wanda's parents were initially resistant to setting a specific date for a home visit. The reason became clear when discussions with their therapist revealed the discomfort they felt about the appearance of their home. A home visit finally took place on the heels of the Christmas holiday. In anticipation of the scheduled visit, a new bed had been purchased for

Wanda. This signaled a significant shift in family sleeping arrangements. There was no longer a need for Wanda to share a bed with her younger brother. Furthermore, Wanda's parents moved their sleeping quarters from the livingroom davenport to their own bedroom. As they showed us around, the family seemed pleased to tell us about these changes, even though their apartment still looked quite drab and barren. The parents' increasing concern about their child's cognitive development was also in evidence in the display of Christmas gifts, which had been selected to encourage their children's social and educational growth.

The anticipation of a home visit was effective in mobilizing Wanda's parents to make important changes in their family life. On another level, the home visit mobilized us to discuss Wanda's relatively barren environmental circumstances with other staff members, thus enabling them to join in a collective effort to provide stimulating and meaningful learning experiences that would broaden this child's experiential base. Field trips were planned, books selected, and appropriate activities planned. As a result, conversations with Wanda began to focus more consciously on topics that could broaden her basic awareness of everyday realities and develop her language skills.

DISCUSSION

Although we are convinced of the value of visits with clients in such naturalistic settings, anxieties and resistances are aroused when there is a departure from the usual approach. This phenomenon has been recognized by various investigators. In a training program for psychiatric residents described by Schwartz, Waldron, and Tidd (1960), many jokes were made when home visiting was introduced as an expectation of staff and residents. Besides the defensive use of humor, there was a tendency to raise questions regarding the value of these assignments, to express objections about busy schedules, and to complain about the new demands being imposed. Behrens and Ackerman (1956) alluded to similar resistances in a mental health clinic, where psychotherapists felt apprehensive about entering their patients' environments. Home visiting was seen as a threat to the family, an invasion of privacy, and a complicating factor in transference behavior.

Resistance to observing and interacting with children in their own home may appear, for some, to be realistic and appropriate at first glance. Upon closer scrutiny, however, it may reveal underlying anxieties and defensive feelings. Although these resistances tend to diminish with experience, their very presence in professionally trained individuals serves as a reminder that unfamiliar settings and situations may also evoke anxieties within patients who, similarly, must approach unfamiliar offices and individuals for help. Moving beyond this recognition through the use of home visits, Fisch (1964) reported that it is possible to provide a "model of flexibility" and an "undefensive approach" for the patient who is similarly threatened by new and unfamiliar experiences. Although home visiting often, admittedly, was approached by Dr. Fisch with trepidation, this feeling was frequently replaced by a sense of mastery. He attributed this feeling to a redefinition of himself as a person who could be less defensive and who could perceive the family as collaborators in a common effort.

Further contributions made by home visits are the added perspectives they provide on the total family profile, exposing both strengths and weaknesses. One family consciously saw a visit by us as an opportunity to demonstrate areas of normalcy, in contrast to the conflicts and turmoil portrayed in therapy hours. This aspect of the home visit has also been emphasized by Satir and Jackson (1961). They stressed the importance of seeing the sick person in dimensions of health as well as illness and the way in which this awareness could be facilitated through home visits. They stressed the dreariness and hopelessness of some diagnostic pictures and the potential for balancing this one-sided perspective by visiting a patient's home, where family members may reveal unsuspected abilities to relate, share humor, or show basic gestures of kindness to one another. On the other hand, it is also possible for an individual or family to present a "façade of adjustment" (Friedman, 1962) that might be penetrated by observing them in their own familiar environment. Friedman describes the observer in a home as having an opportunity to "experience directly the emotional climate of the home and to see through the façade to the underlying, unverbalized family problems" (pp. 133–134).

CONCLUSION

The Day Care Center has been affected in numerous specific ways as a result of the home visits described here. Of major importance has been an increased emphasis in developing a better understanding of each child's environmental context. As a result, treatment efforts have become more focused, realistic, and considerate of each family member. A greater awareness of the existence and needs of family members not in treatment sometimes serves to promote further direct involvement of these individuals in the treatment process.

Because of the recognized value of direct observation in the families' homes, observations of children within their community school also took on greater meaning and significance. School visits included observations of children in their classrooms, lunchrooms, and/or playground activities. These observations contributed additional diagnostic impressions that pointed to new directions and greater clarity in treatment planning.

In some instances, periodic home visits became a part of the regular course of a child's treatment. In those instances, home visits provided valuable assessments of change and progress. Further use of home visiting occurred when a follow-up study was initiated. These contacts became one means of evaluating the current functioning of former patients and served to supplement and clarify data secured through other formal interviewing procedures. Over the years, clinical visits have continued to be an important part of our clinical assessment procedures and treatment for many of the children enrolled at our center.

A variety of training and teaching programs exists within the Day Care Center. Staff members and students in the fields of education, psychiatry, psychology, and social work frequently cross discipline lines. Participating in activities not ordinarily associated with their customary roles enabled them to develop greater understanding and support for their collaboration. Whereas the original purpose for visiting families in their own home setting was related primarily to improving diagnostic and treatment services, it became apparent that other aspects of the program were affected positively as well.

REFERENCES

Behrens, M. L., & Ackerman, N. W. (1956). The home visit as an aid in family diagnosis and therapy. *Social Casework, 37,* 11–19.

Fisch, R. (1964). Home visits in a private psychiatric practice. *Family Process, 3,* 114–126.

Friedman, A. S. (1962). Family therapy as conducted in the home. *Family Process, 1,* 132–140.

Norris-Shortle, C., & Cohen, R. R. (1987). Home visits revisited. *Social Casework, 68,* 54–58.

Satir, V., & Jackson, D. (1961). A review of psychiatric developments in family diagnosis and family treatment. In N. W. Ackerman, F. L. Beatman, & S. N. Sherman (Eds.), *Exploring the base for family therapy* (pp. 29–51). New York: Family Service Association.

Schwartz, D. A., Waldron, R., & Tidd, C. W. (1960). Use of home visits for psychiatric evaluation: Clinical and teaching aspects. *Archives of General Psychiatry, 3,* 57–65.

Spiegel, J. P., & Bell, N. W. (1959). The family of the psychiatric patient. In A. Silvano (Ed.), *American handbook of psychiatry* (Vol. 1; pp. 114–149). New York: Basic Books.

Woods, L. J. (1988). Home-based family therapy. *Social Work, 33,* 211–214.

4

Standby

A Crisis Intervention Program

GORDON K. FARLEY

INTRODUCTION

The most common reason for referral of children to day psychiatric treatment is because of their aggressive and disruptive behaviors. An important part of any successful day treatment program must be a system and plan for the management, control, and change of these behaviors. Treatment settings are more likely to fail in their treatment of children because they cannot control and change the aggressive behaviors of the children than because they cannot understand and educate them. We have used a variety of approaches to deal with aggressive behaviors. We use contingency management, a favorable adult to child ratio, interesting and varied activities, and highly motivating materials. An additional approach to the management of these kinds of problems that has been used in our setting is called *Standby*. Standby has been a part of the Day Care Center program since its beginning in 1962. In the following pages, the reader will find information about the mechanics of our Standby system, including reasons that children are sent to Standby, the steps of a Standby interview, and methods of dealing with children in Standby. An example of an actual Standby is detailed, and there is some discussion of our concerns about Standby.

GORDON K. FARLEY • The Day Care Center, Department of Psychiatry, University of Colorado Health Sciences Center, Denver, Colorado 80262.

OUR STANDBY SYSTEM

The name *Standby* arose from the fact that a staff member is "standing by" to deal with calls from other staff members who feel it appropriate to use this method in situations of classroom disruption or when a child is in acute emotional distress. At one point in our history, we referred to the Standby person as the "Standby officer." We began to realize that this has a legalistic, militaristic ring to it, and revised the name to "Standby person" (SP). During all hours of our operation, an SP is available to deal with calls from staff members who feel that a child needs some individual help. Very soon after their arrival at the Day Care Center, our children are oriented as to the purpose of Standby. We let them know that there is a person available to help them at all times, and we encourage them to ask for a Standby if they need it. We try to establish that Standby is not punishment but is a form of emergency help.

Reasons for Children Being Sent to Standby

There are many reasons for children being sent to Standby, but the large majority of them involve behaviors on the part of the child that are disturbing to the other children or the adults in our setting. This section from our *Standby Manual* will detail and give brief examples of some of the more common reasons.

1. *Physically aggressive—in control.* This may be manifest by a child pushing or bumping against other children or adults in a manipulative or provocative manner. The child is usually aware of his or her actions, and his or her behavior appears to be an attention-getting device. This behavior can be interrupted or stopped by an authority figure. Damage to others or property is deliberately produced and usually minimal.

2. *Physically aggressive—out of control.* The child may be flailing about in a wild and indiscriminate manner, throwing or hitting with little or no concern regarding damage to self, others, or property. This behavior is impossible to control verbally at the time of its occurrence.

3. *Verbally aggressive—in control.* The child manifesting this behavior is usually provocative and/or teasing the teacher or other children. The child may be chatting with classmates at inappropriate times, replying with wisecracks to teachers' questions, or making loud asides regarding class or teacher activity. The language used is usually coherent and not obscene nor excessively primitive. This behavior can usually be interrupted by an authority figure at the time of its occurrence.

4. *Verbally aggressive—out of control.* The child is talking or yelling in little or no relationship to ongoing activity or interaction. The child cannot be interrupted or distracted and brought back to the activity at hand.

The child may be screaming loudly, issuing obscenities or primitive or nonsensical verbalizations.

5. *Direct or open control battle.* The child openly refuses to follow instructions given by the teacher or another authority. The child either does this by verbal refusal to obey or failure to follow a command such as "stand up," "open your book," "read to the class," "take your seat."

6. *Child behaving in a passive–aggressive way.* A child who does not directly refuse to follow orders but who alters the activity or bends the rules in a provocative way. Examples are a child who does what is expected but extremely slowly, or who does correct subject assignments but the wrong pages, intentionally, or who moves when told to but goes to the wrong place, or one who is late starting work.

7. *Anxiety or internal conflict that is not acted out in an aggressive or passive–aggressive way interfering with a child's ability to perform (crying, daydreaming, withdrawal, etc.).* The child's passive behavior is such that he or she is unable to continue to function adequately. Although the child is not expressing the feelings through aggressive behavior, he or she is caught up in difficulties and cannot continue to perform the tasks. Examples of this are the child who is unable to concentrate on schoolwork and sits and daydreams or plays quietly with pencils, etc. Another example is the child who is in tears or crying because she or he is thinking about other factors in her or his life and cannot give attention to the work. The child may fidget and be unable to sit still due to internal anxiety. The content of the school tasks might trigger these and other responses. The stimulus might come from events at home prior to school.

8. *Medical complaint.* The child may ask for a Standby because of illness, real or imagined. The request for a medical Standby may be initiated by either the child or the staff member.

9. *Child asks to be sent.* The child initiates the Standby by verbally requesting to go to Standby in order to have an opportunity to talk. Child may ask to talk with his or her own therapist.

10. *Child breaks rule.* The breaking of certain rules may result in a child automatically being sent to Standby. Examples are leaving an area without permission, running away, climbing on the roof, and throwing snowballs.

11. *Sexual behavior.* The child may attempt to involve another child in sexual play, may be involved in autoerotic activity, or may be displaying sexual behavior toward the teacher.

12. *Other.* Reasons for being sent to Standby that do not fit any described category are marked as "other" and are accompanied by a brief explanation.

These behaviors can be directed toward teachers, other staff members, other children, property, and at times the self (Farley, Sadler, Duchesne, Prodoehl, & Weiman, 1973, pp. 2–4).

The Usual Steps in Standby

Following the occurrence of an event such as those just described, a Standby may be called, and the following actions would take place:

1. The teacher or other staff member calls the front office on their intercom saying, "I would like a Standby in room 1K09."
2. The front office person looks at the posted Standby schedule and calls the SP saying, "There is a Standby for you in room 1K09."
3. The SP responds immediately by going to the classroom, and being informed by the teacher about the events leading up to the call.
4. The SP leaves the classroom with the child and goes to either the Standby room or a clinical office for the Standby interview that typically lasts between 10 and 15 minutes. Occasionally it will be either a shorter or longer interview.
5. As soon as control has been reestablished and there has been a sufficient resolution of the problem, the child is returned to the classroom and the SP informs the teacher about the resolution reached.

Methods Used in the Standby Interview

The interview between the SP and the child is based on a Life Space Interview described by Redl (1959). During the interview, the SP attempts to uncover, understand, and help the child to deal more effectively with the major impulses, feelings, thoughts, and fears that were interfering with classroom functioning at the time of referral for Standby.

Many of our twice-weekly staff meetings revolve around the specific role or roles of the SP. In particular, questions emerge about how to intervene with rageful, screaming, assaultive, out-of-control, and destructive children. Because many of the children we treat have conduct disorders, we have felt that it is important that they realize that we have the ability to control and contain them and that they can feel safe in our setting. With a significant number of children, we have noted that a child who has been aggressive and assaultive in a public school setting becomes docile and compliant when we let him or her know that we are not afraid of them and that someone in our setting is able to manage his or her behavior. Many SPs (often women, but at times men) have reasonably decided that they cannot and will not get into a physical battle with a child. In addition to concerns about the antitherapeutic effects of this interaction on the child, there are concerns that the child may not be controllable or that the physical contact may be misinterpreted as sexual. On these occasions, we have arranged for a backup SP to be available. In the case of an aggressive out-of-control boy, the backup SP may be one of the male staff members, often one of our supervising teachers or the head teacher. In the case of a girl, the backup SP may be a female staff member who is a more neutral figure. At times, we also have had inservice training on methods of safely restraining a struggling, rageful, out-of-control child. During discussions, new and old SPs are encouraged to ask for help, to consider new ways of trying to deal with a difficult child, and to learn from another SP who has discovered a way to engage a given child.

Children bring up many matters in Standby. Frequently, important losses of parents, relatives, and pets are uncovered for the first time during a Standby session. Often the SPs are in a position to help the child grieve for the loss, and later alert the teacher or other caller and enlist his or her aid in continuing the work.

Often a series of Standbys is useful in helping a child to begin to work through a problem. A child who is reluctant to see a repetitive maladaptive pattern in her- or himself, may, after interpretation and confrontation from several different adults, begin to see and deal with it. For example, children who feel demeaned by needing to ask for help can be encouraged to try asking, and children who avoid learning situations because of feeling stupid when admitting they did not know something, can be encouraged to admit a lack of knowledge. This can then be a starting point in learning. Standby personnel are encouraged to attempt to form an alliance with the child in order to work through resistances and explore reasons for behaviors. At times, on successive Standbys, a closer and closer approximation to defining a child's central conflictual area can be made. Early sessions often involve only the identification of the child's affect, some acknowledgment of the affect, and some observations of the child's method for expressing it. Later sessions include, at times, explorations of sources of the affect and various transference phenomena surrounding it.

Another type of intervention centers around the usefulness of linking present difficulties and behaviors with past real or perceived experiences. Teachers are often the recipients of irrational behavior, attitudes, and feelings that are the result of parent–child and child–sibling experiences, interactions, and attitudes. Frequently a SP can help a child in sorting out feelings toward the teacher versus feelings toward parental and other figures.

Some typical ways of handling a Standby are described next, both in general and specific terms. The more specific descriptions are taken from our *Standby Manual* (Farley *et al.,* 1973).

Making Reality More Vivid. In this category the SP explores, questions, elicits facts, or confronts the child with facts and affects, points our rules and expectations of the Day Care Center. Clarifying, revealing, labeling one's own affects in response to the child may be included here. "Scott, you say you jumped on the desk because Cal did it. If Cal jumped off the Empire State Building, would you do that too?" This may involve attempting to bring the child's fantasies and inner feelings into line with outer reality. "Steve, I know you're afraid of going into that room with the kiln, but you know very well that it's not on and even if it were, it couldn't possibly burn you, even if you put your hand on it."

Provoking Guilt or Shame, Eliciting Perspective Taking. The SP may be stern, show open disapproval of child's behavior and consciously attempt to provoke guilt or shame, or elicit perspective taking. "Lester, how do you think you would feel if John broke your airplane the way you just broke his?"

Setting Limits—Verbal. The SP makes verbal suggestions and commands and requests that the disturbing behavior stop for more adaptive functioning or states that thoughts and feelings will not be allowed to become action. Examples are: "Don't do that!" "Even though you're angry, I'm not going to allow you to hurt yourself or anyone else." This often involves accepting the impulse but not allowing the current mode of expression.

Setting Limits—Physical. When the child is out of control, he or she may be restrained or held to prevent him or her from acting out destructive or harmful impulses.

Ventilation. The SP encourages meaningful, appropriate verbalization of affects. "You must feel sad about your father moving out of the house."

Quiet Time—Punitive. The SP isolates the child in an attempt to punish him or her. "I want you to sit there and shut up, and I don't want to hear a word out of you. I'll tell you when it's time to move."

Quiet Time—Cooling Off. The SP reduces stimuli to allow child to regain control and may also allow a brief neutral conversation. "I can see you're upset, and I want you to sit there quietly until you can get hold of yourself."

Linking Present Difficulties with Feelings toward Parents or Other Family Members. The SP points out to the child how the feelings or attitudes expressed to the teacher, another staff person, another child, or object are feelings or attitudes that she or he actually intends for parents or other family members. The SP may say to the child, "I think that the anger that you are showing the teacher is anger that you are really feeling toward your mother and belongs to her."

Support, Empathy, or Relationship Building. The SP offers encouragement, emotional support, understanding, or empathy to the child. The SP may state, "I know that you're upset and I understand the reasons for it." The SP may generalize and say that any child in that situation would feel like that, emphasizing the Day Care Center as a helpful setting. "I think you can do the work that you were asked to do."

Medical Checkup. The SP examines or arranges for an examination for the child because of a medical complaint.

Pointing Out Repetitive Maladaptive Behavior Patterns. The SP points out that the child often acts a certain way in a certain situation. The SP may point out that the child always acts stubborn when asked to perform or always slows down when asked to hurry. The SP may offer alternative ways of expressing feelings. "We've noticed that whenever you get angry at another child, you explode and try to hit him. I wonder if you could show your feelings by telling him how mad you are."

Encouraging the Child to Put Aside Disruptive Thoughts, Impulses, and Feelings. The SP acts in a verbally authoritative way and lets the child know that although he or she may be having disruptive and intrusive aggressive or sexual thoughts or fantasies, that the SP wants the child to put these out of mind for the time being and attend to the task at hand. "Charles, I know that those thoughts about being under the sea, with monsters attacking you, are bothering you a lot, but you're in school now, and I want you to put those thoughts out of your mind and attend to your work."

Other, Such as Mimicking, Persuasion, Negotiation, Rewarding, Use of Humor, etc. This category includes ways of handling Standby that do not fit in any of the other categories. Included in this category may be mimicking the child to show how he or she is acting, helping the child to rehearse new and alternative behaviors, contracting with the child, or writing a note to a teacher, parent, therapist, or another child. The SP may offer to compromise with the child around an issue or offer a reward for good behavior.

Standby Records

From very early in our history, we have kept some form of daily log sheets to record information about Standby incidents. These records are

Child's name:
Date: Time: (from_____to_____)
Sender: Requested by child?   Medical?
Reason for being sent and contributing factors (if known):
Intervention:
Resolution:
Medication given: Time: Dosage:

_____

Signature, degree, staff position

Figure 1. Standby Report Form.

primarily used to communicate to other team members; however, they also help provide clinical material for staff discussions of individual children and have been a source of a naturalistic clinical research study (Sadler & Blom, 1970). One early form of log sheet was designed by a Standby committee headed by the author. It showed the date, time of day, part of the program involved, specific situation of separation (such as day before or after holiday, day before or after absence, etc.), name and discipline of referring agent, reason for child being sent, method of handling the Standby, name and discipline of the SP, whether it was a group or individual Standby, and duration of the Standby episode. On these log sheets, there was also a space for a narrative written account of reasons for the child being sent and the methods of handling the Standby. In our ongoing review of the use of Standby in our setting, it became apparent that the form we were using was too extensive, cumbersome, and time consuming to fill out. Little use of the forms was being made after their completion, and only about one-half of the encounters were being recorded. A committee looked into the matter, and the result was a new streamlined form that recorded only the time, the name of the child, the name of the sender, the name of the SP, the reasons for the Standby, and the intervention and resolution. Compliance has reached over 95%. An example of our new form is shown in Figure 1.

The Standby Person and Standby Training

Child psychiatrists, child psychologists, social workers, secretaries, administrative officers, medical students, nursing students, psychiatry residents, child psychiatry fellows, psychology interns, graduate teachers, staff teachers, and social work students have all, at times, served as SPs. Early in the training year, new SPs are oriented to the procedures and practices of Standby over several 1-hour sessions by our Standby coordinator, Caroline Corkey. The overall purpose and philosophy, the development of Standby in the Day Care Center, and different methods of handling Standby are presented and discussed.

Over the many years we have used Standby, we have accumulated a library of videotapes that demonstrate faculty and staff members in a variety of Standby situations. These tapes are shown to new SPs followed by discussion about what to do in ambiguous and anxiety-provoking situations. During these discussions, suggestions come from both new and old SPs, and an atmosphere of give and take, willingness to reveal mistakes, and mutual learning is established. New SPs are then offered the opportunity to observe Standby interviews of veteran SPs for a 2-week period. Following this intense orientation, they are then expected to do Standbys on their own with supervision available. Standby events often are discussed during individual trainee supervision and are useful in bringing to the front important issues of interpersonal relationships and clinical practice.

AN EXAMPLE OF A STANDBY

Many examples could be given both of successful and less than successful resolutions in Standby. The following is a condensed example of a relatively successful Standby:

At 9:15 A.M. the SP was called by Mr. G. When the SP got to the classroom, he was told that Sheri had come in about 10 minutes late to school this morning and seemed very rushed. When Mr. G. asked her to do some arithmetic problems, she got very angry at him, screamed, called him an old goat, said that the problems were too hard and that she wouldn't *do them for him*. When he encouraged her to give them a try, she said that she hated him because he never helped her, was spending all his time helping the other kids, and that she never got her share of his help. Mr. G. told the SP that he felt that since Sheri's anger was so disproportionate to the event, and apparently unprovoked, her feelings probably had something to do with some things that had happened at home. The SP suggested that Sheri come with him to his office to talk about the difficulty she and Mr. G. were having and she angrily agreed. The conversation in the office went something like this:

> *SP:* Can you tell me what happened between you and Mr. G. in the class-room just now?
> *Sheri:* Well, he was making me do this work and I didn't want to. I hate the old goat. He never gives me any help, he's always helping the other kids. He makes me do work that's too hard for me. Sometimes he gives me the wrong

answers and confuses me. I won't do any work for him when he won't help me at all and spends all his time with the other kids.

SP: How did you feel when you came to school this morning?

Sheri: I was really mad. My mother didn't get up in time to fix me any breakfast, so she didn't give me any, and I was hungry when I got to school, and I was really mad. Besides that, last night my mother had two candy bars and gave them both to my brother, David. He always gets more than I do; besides, my mother always spends more time with him than she does with me.

SP: Sounds like the same thing goes on here at school, doesn't it?

Sheri: What do you mean?

SP: Well, it sounds to me as though you kind of feel that Mr. G. isn't giving you anything, and is giving the other kids everything and spending time with them just the way your mother didn't give you breakfast and gave both candy bars to David and spends more time with him.

Sheri: It really made me mad when she did that. She never gives me any breakfast. I was still mad when I got to school.

SP: It sounds to me as if you were showing some of your feelings to Mr. G. that your mother really deserved to get.

Sheri: Yeah. I was mad at my mother and taking it out on Mr. G.

SP: That's right. Do you think you could go back to class and work now.

Sheri: I guess so.

The SP took Sheri back to the classroom, explained briefly to Mr. G. what happened in the Standby, and Sheri went back to work.

RESERVATIONS ABOUT STANDBY

At times, we consider the abandonment of the Standby program. The organization and maintenance of the program is a major effort for one of our faculty members. The covering of approximately 30 hours per week of clinical time represents a major outlay of professional time. We depend heavily on people in training to fill the gaps. Many of our trainees arrive in September and leave in late April. There are times when the permanent staff is stretched very thin. During certain times of the year (before and after holidays, for example), there is heavy use of Standby, and several Standbys may be called simultaneously. Staff burn-out on Standby is not uncommon. When this occurs, we attempt to adapt by increasing the classroom personnel, putting on a backup SP, or re-evaluating the program structures. Each time cessation is considered, we are reminded of the usefulness of the service by the teachers, aides, and other staff members. The usefulness of the training experience for those in a number of disciplines is also brought to our attention, and many remember Standby as the high point in their training.

REFERENCES

Farley, G. K., Sadler, J. E., Duchesne, E., Prodoehl, M., & Weiman, E. A. (1973). *A Standby Manual for the Day Care Center.* Unpublished manuscript, University of Colorado Health Sciences Center, Denver.

Redl, F. (1959). Strategy and techniques of the life space interview. *American Journal of Orthopsychiatry, 29,* 1–18.

Sadler, J., & Blom, G. E. (1970). Standby: A clinical research study of child deviant behavior in a psychoeducational setting. *Journal of Special Education, 4,* 89–103.

5

The Role of Education in Our Day Treatment Program

SARA GOODMAN ZIMET and RALPH IMHOFF

THE FRAMEWORK FOR OTHER TREATMENT COMPONENTS

Schooling for the 23 children at the Day Care Center is a primary component of their therapeutic program. The school day begins at 8:45 in the morning and continues through 2:30 in the afternoon, 5 days a week, and provides the framework within which the milieu functions.

Most of the 6 hours the children are at the center each day is spent with their teacher and assistant teacher in their classrooms, participating primarily but not solely in group-oriented activities. There are four classroom groups with five or six children in each. Most group therapy is classroom based. This focus on the classroom tends to further solidify the children's identification with it as their home base at the center.

With the exception of lunch and free play before and during school hours, children are almost always with their group mates. Lunch takes 30 minutes, from 12:00 to 12:30, during which time the children are likely to sit with children other than those from their classroom and with adult supervisors other than their teachers. The exception to this rule is for children who are at an early developmental level in their ability to handle changes in routine. Thus in order to minimize the disruption that inevitably occurs when these young children move to another room in the building and are placed with adults with whom they infrequently

SARA GOODMAN ZIMET and RALPH IMHOFF • The Day Care Center, Department of Psychiatry, University of Colorado Health Sciences Center, Denver, Colorado 80262.

interact, either their teacher or teacher–assistant eats lunch with them in the lunchroom. (For a complete description of the lunch and other food programs at the Center, see the chapter by Zimet and Schultz.)

The other predictable time that a child may go to another room is during his or her therapy sessions. The children's individual therapists—speech therapists and psychotherapists—pick them up and bring them back to the classroom one to two times a week for approximately 30 minutes at a time.

CHARACTERISTICS OF OUR SCHOOL ENVIRONMENT

Theoretical Background

Our school curriculum is based on a number of parallel theoretical positions: (a) the cognitive developmental perspective of Jean Piaget (1970); (b) the educational and psychological pragmatism of John Dewey (1938) and Carl Rogers (1983); (c) the psychodynamic understanding and developmental perspectives of Anna Freud (1946) and Erik Erikson (Midcentury White House Conference on Children and Youth, 1966); and (d) the contingency management approach of Bandura (1969, 1986), Patterson and his colleagues (1976, 1982), and Skinner (1974). Our program emphasizes presenting children with experiences and material that are appropriate to their developmental level of functioning in each of the domains of their lives (e.g., cognitive, affective, and social). We recognize that children need to confirm reality and increase the meaningfulness of their educational experiences through their own senses by the active manipulation of their environment. We also recognize the role of unconscious conflict and transference manifestations in the teaching and learning process. Furthermore, our program acknowledges the importance of a predictable structure of the daily environment and of the content of teaching materials. We are keenly aware of the importance of a feedback loop in communications between teacher and pupil and of the impact of perceived competence and self-esteem on children's academic performance and social behavior. Our staff members firmly believe that, barring any severe organic interference, the children are capable of learning material that is presented in interesting, well-organized, and developmentally appropriate contexts.

Proven Practices

There are certain characteristics of public schools that have been systematically associated with fostering high self-esteem, promoting social and scholastic success, and reducing the likelihood of emotional and behavioral disorders in children. In these schools, the adults present themselves as good models of behavior. They show respect for the students, and their expectations of the students' behavior and academic performance are set at appropriately high levels. Children are given the opportunity to take responsibility for and to participate in the running of their lives at school. Discipline is based on setting clear and reasonable expectations within a context of praise and encouragement. There is sparing use of punishment. On the other hand, the children are not protected from the natural consequences of their behavior, although they are protected from serious risk. We feel that they learn a great deal from guided discovery of the impact of their actions. In other words, these real life occurrences are used as therapeutic opportunities for developing new perceptions about old behaviors and new ways of dealing with old problems. Discipline also is maintained within the classroom by (a) getting into activities quickly with a minimum of start-up time; (b) creating a daily structure that is clear and predictable; (c) teaching in a class-based versus individual-based mode; (d) giving clear and unambiguous feedback to the children on their performance; and (e) using praise generously for good performance. These techniques have been shown to minimize the incidence of disciplinary problems and the need for disciplinary interventions. Schools with children who manifest high levels of problem behaviors tend to be more authoritarian, with an emphasis on harsh and strict (often petty) rule enforcement rather than on the encouragement of learning. In addition, staff members tend to isolate themselves from both the children and parents. (For a more complete review of this line of research, see Wolkind & Rutter, 1985.) Successful schools, in effect, combine firmness, warmth, high expectations, and a practical approach to teaching.

We believe that a similar educational atmosphere can be created, with appropriate modifications, to meet the needs of children with behavioral and emotional disorders, and this is what we have done. In other words, although the curriculum contains similar domains to those found in most public schools, the hierarchical arrangement and degree of emphasis within these domains are likely to differ. For example, where academic areas head the list in the public schools, emotional and social learning are likely to have top priority in our school program. Furthermore, where the child's safety and security may be taken for granted in most public schools, our behavior management interventions are thoughtfully and consistently applied; each child quickly learns that he or she and all of his or her peers are in a safe environment. We also feel that such an environment is consistent with other parts of the program. In this regard we present the children and their families with a consistent and coherent treatment program.

Curriculum Characteristics

Our School Curriculum Is Integrated and Functional. Learning in one area of the children's lives is connected to other areas of their lives, either naturally or from a conscious effort to teach this connection. Although separate skill areas may be taught occasionally, they are always integrated into the fabric of the children's lives in the classroom. It is a functional curriculum because *what* they are taught is relevant to their immediate daily lives, and *how* they are taught prepares them for future learning. In contrast to earlier beliefs that children with emotional disorders were incapable of learning until they had been cured of their disorders, we believe that these children are capable of engaging in the learning process and that they will become active learners when placed in an environment where active learning is expected of them. In effect, academic, social, and physical skills are expected to develop at the same time that they are being treated for their emotional and/or behavioral disorders.

We believe that an integrated and functional curriculum addresses pertinent matters that affect the children's relationships with their peers and the significant adults in their lives, as well as concerns that are of interest to the broader community and to society. These issues have both negative and positive valences. For example, we have had children in our program with unusual health problems, such as hemophilia, sickle-cell anemia, asthma, immunological disorders, and epilepsy. In addition to providing inservice training for our staff, we draw up guidelines for discussing these issues with the other children as a way of preventing risks to the ill child and increasing the competency of the children as a group in dealing with emergencies that may come up. In like manner, we deal with emotionally loaded news items of local and national concern, such as kidnapping, physical, sexual, and substance abuse, race and gender bias, disease epidemics, and the threat of a nuclear holocaust. In a more positive vein, we also recognize and celebrate the usual holidays and attend to local and national elections. (See the chapter by Lee for examples of how this teacher uses these occasions in the curriculum.)

The Curriculum Is Child-Centered. It is tailored to the characteristics of the children. For example, our experience with and research about these children indicates that they are egocentric, wrapped in concerns about themselves, and unable to imagine beyond their immediate circumstances. Most lack basic social skills, such as making and keeping friends and behaving appropriately in public. They have difficulty in generalizing from one situation to another and in transferring the skills learned in one setting to other settings. Their repertoire of behaviors is limited, and there appears to be an unwillingness to try new approaches and to even consider alternative strategies. Their judgments about their own affective state and work performance tend to be inaccurate and at odds with the estimates held by objective others, such as their teachers and psychotherapists (Zimet & Farley, 1986). Instruction begins at the child's developmental level, at the level of his or her immediate concern—from "me" to "them"—beginning with the familiar and gradually moving to the unfamiliar, using what Bruner (1960) has described as the *spiral curriculum*. Academic learning and associated activities are organized to coincide with the child's developmental level and to expand horizontally and then vertically as the child is ready to do so. (Examples of this approach are described in "The People-to-People Travel Project" and in "The Structure and Function of the Human Body" in the chapter by Parsons and Imhoff, "Special Projects.")

The Curriculum Is Balanced. It includes physical activities, both structured (i.e., swimming) and unstructured but supervised (i.e., free play), interspersed with seatwork (e.g., listening to cassettes, writing, and reading), and other quiet or concentrated work activities. The following is an example of a typical day's schedule for each of our classroom groups by stage of development (see the discussion of the Developmental Therapy Objectives Rating Form (DTORF) later):

All Groups

    8:45– 9:00 Supervised play in the gym or playground.
    9:00– 9:15 Morning snack in the cafeteria.
    9:15–12:00 See schedules listed later.
    12:00–12:30 Lunch in the cafeteria.
    12:30– 2:30 See schedules listed later.
    2:30   Leave for home.

On Thursday afternoons, all of the classroom groups go to a neighborhood swimming pool where they receive swimming instruction.

Stages I/II Children

    9:15– 9:45 Warm-up for the day and talk time.
    9:45–10:45 Language arts (e.g., TV viewing of "Sesame Street" with
               follow-up activities and work with the computer). On
               Monday only, group therapy between 10:00 and 10:30.

10:45–11:00 Supervised play in the playground.
12:30– 1:00 Kitchen cleanup.
 1:00– 1:30 Science and math content and skill building.
 1:30– 2:00 Structured play time.
 2:00– 2:15 Games and music.
 2:15– 2:30 Review of the day in preparation for leaving.

Stage III Children

 9:15– 9:30 Warm-up for the day and talk time.
 9:30–10:00 Language arts (e.g., journal writing with optional sharing of entry with class and work with the computer).
10:00–10:45 Mathematics activities.
10:45–11:15 Supervised play in the playground.
11:15–12:00 Reading with a partner or practicing math skills.
12:30–12:50 Language arts (e.g., handwriting and literature).
12:50– 1:45 Reading workbooks or special integrated language arts activities (e.g., writing stories and reports, or carrying out science, social studies, or art projects).
 1:45– 2:10 Supervised play in the playground (Wednesday only, group speech therapy between 1:30 and 2:15).
 2:10– 2:30 Sustained silent reading and checkout story books to take home.

Stage IV Children

 9:15– 9:45 Warm-up for the day and talk time.
 9:45–10:30 Mathematics instruction and activities with and without the computer.
10:30–11:00 Reading and writing instruction and activities with and without the computer.
11:00–11:45 Supervised playground activities.
11:45–12:00 Prepare for lunch.
12:30– 1:30 Language arts instruction and activities (Wednesday only, group speech therapy).
 1:30– 2:00 Supervised playground activities.
 2:00– 2:30 Review of the day in preparation for leaving.

Dealing with Transitions

Transitions are anticipated and are handled with sensitivity and careful planning. Initially we are concerned about the transitions that occur when the children first enter our program and then when they move from one activity to another within their classrooms. We also are alert to the difficulties they experience when they move from their classrooms to another setting within the center (e.g., to the playground and the lunchroom). Traveling to the swimming pool one afternoon each week and going on occasional field trips associated with "play" (e.g., to the circus and stock show) or specific scholarly projects (e.g., to the zoo and museum of natural history) present another challenge because these transitions involve locations away from the center. Major transitions occur when their therapists leave and new ones are assigned and when they move from our school to one in the community. This latter one involves interagency communication and cooperation and a great deal of planning with the children and their families (see "Ending Day Treatment: Let's Talk About It," in the chapter, "Special Projects," by Parsons and Imhoff).

Group Placement, Educational Planning, and Monitoring Progress

Although the primary focus of instruction is the group (or *towards* the group for the youngest children), individual educational plans (IEPs) are formulated using a developmental assessment instrument, the Developmental Therapy Objectives Rating Form (DTORF) (Wood, Combs, Gunn, & Weller, 1986). The DTORF taps four domains: "Behavior, Communication, Socialization and Academics, with items ranging from very basic and low level behaviors at the awareness level to very complex behaviors reflecting high levels of integrated, coordinated social and cognitive activity" (p. 46). The objectives are sequenced into five separate stages of development, each representing a distinct level, Stage 1 is the lowest and Stage 5 is the highest. The DTORF is first completed by the teacher during the child's 2- to 3-week evaluation in order (a) to get a baseline measure; (b) to determine in which classroom the child should be placed; and (c) to construct the IEP. Ratings also are done by the teachers three times a year throughout the child's treatment, in order to measure and document each child's progress.

Once an area for learning has been identified that will capture the interests of the children in the group, a range of specific activities are planned that have embedded within them the skills that the children need to learn, both social and academic (e.g., cooperation, communication, and measurement). We tend to overplan activities so that unexpected events (i.e., a broken projector, a flat tire, or a new opportunity) may be handled smoothly. Throughout the process, evaluation plays a very important role, for both the children and the teacher. It involves multiple perspectives including personal reflections and feedback from peers and others.

THE ROLE OF OUR TEACHERS

Their Attitudes and Behaviors

We believe that the teachers' attitudes and behaviors are among the most crucial elements in the therapeutic educational process because the teachers spend more time with the children than any other staff member. Therefore, all of our teachers are highly trained professionals with much experience teaching and working with children who have emotional and behavioral disturbances. Although some mental health professionals have advocated a more active role for the teacher (LaVietes, 1962), we believe that it is important to clearly define the primary role of each of our staff members by their discipline and training. The teacher is primarily responsible for creating a therapeutic classroom environment that will facilitate each child's ability to learn. Therefore, she or he is expected to find a balance between detached concern and overinvolvement in the children's emotional problems (Mumford, 1968). In practical terms, when a child *persists* in expressing his or her conflicts in the classroom, the teacher is expected to direct the child toward attending to school-related matters and to deal with other problem areas through other channels: (a) immediately with a "Standby" person (see the chapter by Farley describing this intervention), and/or (b) at her or his next psychotherapy session. If a child reveals important therapy-related material to the teacher, she or he is expected to relay this to the team with the child's knowledge. The child or parent's therapist then may wish to pursue the matter at the next therapy session.

In effect, our teachers are aware that emotional problems are likely to interfere with a child's ability to pay attention and to learn, but they are also aware of the many resources available to the child to work on those problems while carrying out his or her work as children. In a parallel way, our teachers recognize that, at times, their own personal issues may interfere in their work with the children, the children's parents, and with other staff members. They are expected to work with other mental health professionals on a team as "experts" in their field and to be able to ask for help from other experts. They need to differentiate between asking for help as a personal defeat and using another person as a resource, just as they would expect the children they teach to use resources outside themselves.

Encouraging Professional and Personal Development

To facilitate the recognition of this parallel process, the teachers receive clinical–educational supervision on a regularly scheduled basis. This means, in effect, that they are helped to understand the contributions they make to the smooth running of a healthy system, as well as to the problems of a troubled system and the impact that either system has on troubled children.

In a therapeutic environment such as ours, there is the temptation for the supervisor to assume the role of the teacher's therapist. Although we believe that it is important for the supervisor to be supportive of a teacher during a period of personal stress, we also believe that the teacher should be encouraged by his or her supervisor to seek help for the problem outside the Center. The primary focus of supervision, therefore, should be the teacher's work with the children.

Engaging Parents

Although we do not blame parents for the children's troubles, our teachers are well aware of the complex interaction among family members. They are sensitive to the possibility of being perceived by both the child and parents as the "other parent" and the consequences of these perceptions. For example, the teachers are aware that the same child may treat them at different times as the adored, hated, or wished-for parent and may attempt to reconstruct the family conflicts within the classroom. The teachers also recognize that changes that occur in one system are likely to affect what happens to the children in other systems. Thus our program emphasizes the important role that communication plays among teachers, children, and parents. To this end, regular, frequent contacts with parents are made by daily and/or weekly notes to them, and phone calls, at appropriate times, for transmitting and seeking information and for engaging parents in their children's schooling. The entire team also meets with each child's parents at least once a year to discuss their child's progress and to plan the next year's IEP.

Interfacing with Other Teachers

Under the leadership of the head teacher, a meeting is held once a week with all the center teachers, where they discuss such issues as (a) immediate and long-range plans regarding individual teacher's goals and the center's goals; (b) professional development; and (c) interfacing with other program components.

Interfacing with Other Program Components

As discussed in the chapter by Farley that describes the overall treatment program, the coordinating mechanism of all the treatment components is the team. Each teacher meets with the team, which is made up of all the people working directly with the child and his or her family and a team leader. They each meet once a week for 15 minutes. Team decisions that impact on other staff members' interactions with a child are transmitted by memo.

Opportunities to discuss recent developments and their impact on a child's treatment are provided during staff meetings or at review conferences, where teachers report on the children's life in the classroom. In addition, a year-end summary of each child's progress in the educational program is written by the teacher and is kept in the child's chart along with other documentation (i.e., the IEPs, reports of academic and cognitive testing, and the DTORFs).

DISCREPANCIES BETWEEN WHAT WE SAY AND WHAT WE DO

Just as with other professionals working at the center, if you were to observe the work being done in the classrooms with the statements made in this chapter, you would no doubt be struck by the fact that although each staff member shares a great deal in common with every other staff member, each expresses a clear individuality as well. When such discrepancies are noted between "what we say we do" and "what we actually do," we need to ask ourselves if the discrepancies represent a misunderstanding of the center's goals, aims, and/or philosophical position, or if they are pointing to a change in direction that is beginning to emerge. In either case, it is important to use our observations diagnostically to determine what kind of intervention would be appropriate. It may simply be a topic for discussion during a supervisory session or among the staff at large, or it may require more documentation and discussion during a program planning retreat.

CONCLUSIONS

Schooling for the children at the Day Care Center provides the framework for all the other treatment components of our program. The children identify their classroom group as their home base at the center.

Our school curriculum as well as all the other components of our therapeutic treatment program is built upon a number of parallel theoretical positions represented by John Dewey, Erik Erikson, Anna Freud, Jean Piaget, B. F. Skinner, and others. Consistent with these positions are characteristics of schools that foster high self-esteem, promote social and scholastic success, and reduce the likelihood of emotional disorders. We have attempted to create a curriculum model incorporating these practices in our daily work with the children. Thus our school program is integrated and functional, child-centered and balanced. It combines firmness, warmth, high expectations, and an approach to teaching that is consistent with other parts of our program.

REFERENCES

Bandura, A. (1969). *Principles of behavior modification.* New York: Holt, Rinehart & Winston.

Bandura, A. (1986). *Social foundations of thought and action.* Englewood Cliffs, NJ: Prentice-Hall.

Bruner, J. (1960). *The process of education.* Cambridge: Harvard University Press.

Dewey, J. (1938). *Experience and education.* New York: Macmillan.

Midcentury White House Conference on Children and Youth (1966). A healthy personality for every child. In J. F. Rosenblith & W. Allinsmith (Eds.), *The causes of behavior II: Readings in child development and educational psychology.* Boston: Allyn & Bacon.

Freud, A. (1946). *Psychoanalytical treatment of children.* London: Imago Publishing Co.

Kounin, J. S. (1975). An ecological approach to classroom activity settings: Some methods and findings. In R. A. Weinberg & F. H. Wood (Eds.), *Observation of pupils and teachers in mainstreaming and special education settings: Alternative strategies.* Minneapolis: Leadership Training Institute, University of Minnesota.

LaVietes, R. (1962). The teacher's role in the education of the emotionally disturbed child. *American Journal of Orthopsychiatry, 32,* 854–862.

Mumford, E. (1968). Teacher response to school mental health programs. *American Journal of Psychiatry, 125,* 113–119.

Patterson, G. R. (1976). *Living with children: New methods for parents and teachers.* Champaign, IL: Research Press.

Patterson, G. R., Reid, J. B., Jones, R. R., & Conger, R. E. (1982). *Families with aggressive children* (Vol. 1). Eugene, OR: Castilia Publishing Co.

Piaget, J. (1970). *The science of education and the psychology of the child.* New York: Orion Press.

Rogers, C. (1983). *Freedom to learn: A view of what education might become* (rev. ed.). Columbus, OH: Merrill Publishing Co.

Skinner, B. F. (1974). *About behaviorism.* New York: Alfred A. Knopf.

Swap, S. M., Prieto, A. G., & Hath, R. (1982). Ecological perspectives of the emotionally disturbed child. In R. L. McDowell, G. W. Adamson, & F. H. Woods (Eds.), *Teaching emotionally disturbed children.* Boston: Little, Brown.

Wolkind, S., & Rutter, M. (1985). Sociocultural factors. In M. Rutter & L. Hersov (Eds.), *Child and adolescent psychiatry* (2nd ed.). Boston: Blackwell Scientific Publications.

Wood, M. W., Combs, C., Gunn, A., & Weller, D. (1986). *Developmental therapy in the classroom.* Austin, TX: Pro-ed.

Zimet, S. G., & Farley, G. K. (1986). Four perspectives on the competence and self-esteem of emotionally disturbed children beginning day treatment. *Journal of the American Academy of Child Psychiatry, 25,* 76–83.

Reading and Writing in a Therapeutic Classroom

CAROL L. LEE

A THERAPEUTIC CLASSROOM: ACADEMIC DILEMMAS

Currently in my classroom there are six children: Evelyn, Alan, Bob, Jerry, Ryan, and Tiffany. Not a large number for a classroom, but what a large task ahead of me. Six children, between the ages of 7 and 11 with a variety of emotional difficulties and learning needs. Where shall I begin to teach them? What do they know about reading and writing? More important, what do they feel about reading and writing? In this chapter, I will share with the reader some of my teaching experiences with these children at the Day Care Center.

At the back desk sits Evelyn reading a paperback book about a lost dog. Evelyn is a strong reader, but she has not done well in previous school settings. She is a tall 11-year-old with big blue eyes and a round face. She gazes blankly away from her book and is far away from the classroom in her thoughts. Alan is not content to go unnoticed for very long. He is the wiggly, wise-cracking boy who, though he is just 9, looks like a miniature rebellious teenager with his mod spike haircut and pierced earring. Alan is an average reader, but he avoids assignments involving writing. However, he has just finished a love note that he is delivering to Tiffany, his most recent girlfriend. As he sits down, he

CAROL L. LEE • The Day Care Center, Department of Psychiatry, University of Colorado Health Sciences Center, Denver, Colorado 80262.

turns to joke loudly with Jerry, a large 7-year-old boy with a shy smile and big, dark mischievous eyes. Bob, who has been working diligently in his journal, looks up with annoyance at the interruption. He realizes that he has been left out of the flirting and friendly banter and calls Alan an unflattering name under his breath. Andrew, my half-time aid has pulled up a chair beside Ryan, an immature 10-year-old student with serious reading difficulties. I am grateful to have Andrew—for this is a lively, engaging group of children who challenge me continually with their academic and emotional neediness.

Academic and Social Delays

Most of my students are concerned about falling behind other children their age both academically and socially. They want to be accepted by their peers in their neighborhoods and schools. They may not be fully aware of how much or how little control they have over a given situation in their lives nor the ingredients or sacrifices necessary to change some chronic situations. Still, they and their parents are aware of society's expected match between chronological age and grade levels and the stigma attached to falling behind. Our therapeutic classrooms—with overlapping ages and abilities—are situated outside of the public school setting and can offer a welcome reprieve from these pressures. However, most of our students will return to public schools within 2 to 3 years. For many reasons, including societal pressures, educational rights, and self-esteem, academic delays must be recognized and treated along with the emotional problems that precipitated referral to the Day Care Center.

I occasionally address the issue of reasons for previous academic problems or delays in school achievement both individually and in group discussions with the children. This gives my students a chance to verbalize and understand their concerns. We have briefly explored such possible reasons as chronic absences, hospitalizations, or varying learning disabilities that may have limited their complete control over past school problems. We have also talked about how people can be "absent" from the tasks at hand even when they are in class, if some personal problems are distracting them. At this point in one of our discussions, Evelyn spoke up quite emphatically: "The reason I couldn't keep my mind on my schoolwork was because my mom and dad kept fighting over which one would get custody of me." Indeed, for Evelyn, it had taken over a year for the court to decide the bitter custody battle between her parents—a year that Evelyn had spent angrily in an inpatient unit of a psychiatric hospital. She had often been so uncontrollable after one of her parent's visits to the inpatient unit that she was unable to attend the hospital's school facility on that day. At these times, her face and body often showed her anger; her voice was high pitched and whiny, and her handwriting was so illegible that she was referred to occupational therapy for fine motor problems. When the custody battle was finally resolved, Evelyn left the hospital to live with her father and was placed in our day treatment center. The new stability brought calm and confidence to Evelyn that began to show in the steady progress she made in all her academic subjects. Her penmanship was remarkably neater and legible, her oppositionality had lessened, and smiles began to re- place her angry frown.

Multiple Problems, Multiple Causes

Although Evelyn's emotional and academic problems may seem clearly related to her parents' difficult situation, it is more likely that an interaction of many factors contributes to the school problems of children in our center. In Evelyn's case, oppositional personality, parent loss issues (in addition to the divorce, she had been adopted as an infant), chronic school absences, poor peer relationships, low self-esteem, and lack of success at her previous school setting are additional symptoms or factors of emotional disturbance that contributed to her school problems. In effect, at our center, it is recognized that there are many reasons for the children's poor academic performance, and these reasons are usually complex ones involving the interaction of two or more factors. As a teacher working with children who have multiple problems, it is only natural to wonder about causes of academic failure and to hypothesize about them. I have become cautious not to oversimplify the complex dynamics occurring in the low-achieving child with severe emotional problems. A diagnosis of a specific reading disability presents a particular set of dilemmas. Ryan and Bob, who are described next, are examples of children with both primary learning and emotional problems.

Living with Learning Disabilities

A deeply disturbed and immature boy, Ryan, at age 10, is still basically a nonreader. He struggles to read at a middle first-grade level. Prior to entering my classroom, an outside evaluation diagnosed Ryan as having dyslexia. The report described him as having a specific reading disability involving significant deficits in language, short-term memory, and auditory phonetic processing. Intellectual testing showed him to be of average intelligence. All of this information was very important for him and his family to hear because he had come to think of himself as stigmatized as mentally retarded.

However, like many of us, Ryan had difficulty interpreting the implications of such a diagnosis as dyslexia (often referred to as specific reading disability) to his continuing work in school. This is illustrated by his comments to me just a few days after entering my class. He told me he could not be expected to do a simple assignment I had given him, because he said, "My brain doesn't work right—it's all mixed up." He went on to explain that this was why he could not remember the sounds of the letters (which was not, however, the task on this assignment). He seemed relieved to tell me about his condition, which gave us an opportunity to discuss privately his feelings about reading at a later time. Ryan's explanation of his dyslexia revealed an oversimplification of the total reading process and did not include how years of failure in school, immaturity, dependence, and other serious emotional problems had complicated this diagnosis.

Of course children react differently to information shared with them about learning disabilities. Bob had long-standing emotional and language problems and a history of abuse and neglect. After several foster home placements, Bob had still been in diapers and sucking on a bottle at age 4 when he was adopted by a loving family. But his emotional problems were so debilitating that he could not function in the public schools. He was extremely anxious, oppositional, and aggressive. He entered our program when he was 8 years old. By the time Bob arrived in my classroom at age 10 he had made much progress but had been diagnosed with dyslexia. The term *dyslexia* was new to Bob and his parents. Bob was determined to prove to me, his new teacher, that he did not have dyslexia—that nothing was "wrong" with him. Currently he works very hard at his desk in all his assignments but resists any tutoring efforts that make him look or feel different from the other kids. Originally he avoided writing, but now he has come to enjoy expressing himself in writing, so much that he writes several pages in his journal almost every day.

Unlike Bob's determined personality, Ryan's immaturity, dependency on teachers, and fear of making mistakes are hindering his academic progress. Even with such different personalities and different reactions to being labeled *learning disabled,* I feel both boys have experienced secondary emotional problems as the result of prolonged reading delays and perceived humiliation in front of peers. The gap between themselves and their classmates will most likely become even more noticeable as they continue in school. Motivating children with learning disabilities to continue to risk to learn in spite of a slower progress than their classmates is a formidable challenge for teachers, especially teachers of children who experience primary emotional difficulties also.

ENGAGING CHILDREN IN READING: BOOKS, BOOKS, AND MORE BOOKS

Perspectives and Priorities

In planning ways to engage children in the reading process it is important to keep in mind the children's perspectives on reading. I am reminded of a class discussion that illustrates this point: A "Reading Is Fundamental" (RIF) book distribution was about to take place in our center, during which each child could select two paperback books to keep. First, we talked about the meaning of the phrase, "Reading Is Fundamental" and the reasons why it was important to be able to read. Next, we talked about another phrase from the RIF program, "Reading Is Fun." Although most agreed that it was fun to hear stories read to them and that it felt good to be able to read by themselves, reading was not always fun. They went on to tell me when it was not fun for them, such as when (a) the words were too hard to figure out; (b) the words were too easy or did not make any sense; (c) people laughed at them or made fun of the way they read; and (d) no one would read a book with them or listen to them read.

Learning what is important to my students helps me keep a focus on priorities in planning for reading activities. One such priority is the enjoyment of sharing a book together that is done in several ways in our classroom. Sometimes I choose a book to read in front of the whole class. Classics such as *Call It Courage* (Sperry, 1940) and *Charlotte's Web* (White, 1952), or more modern, humorous tales such as *Bunnicula* (Howe & Howe, 1979), are class favorites.

Another enjoyable way to share books is to sit next to a child and share a book he or she has chosen from the stacks of books around the room. This gives an added opportunity to individually reinforce important concepts, especially for the beginning reader. At the back of our classroom is a big orange couch. Usually only two or three people sit on the couch at one time because it is easier to see the pictures and because a child can get more individual reading practice time. But at times we have *all* squeezed together on that big couch to take turns reading such favorites as *The Ugly Duckling* (Parnell, 1987a) or *The Little Red Hen* (Parnell, 1987b).

Choosing Predictable Books

After recess when it is Partners Time, two children may choose to either practice math flash cards or read a book together or do both if they have time. Usually the pile of flash cards goes untouched. The favorite books that are often chosen are "predictable books." A predictable book is one in which children can quickly begin to predict what the author is going to say and how it will be said. *Fortunately* (Charlip, 1964) is an example of a book that children delight in guessing what will happen on the next page. Repetitive patterns, rhyming, rhythm of the language, and familiarity of the story structure are other characteristics of predictable books (Rhodes, 1981). Rhyming and riddle books, simple folk tales, and stories with repeated lines such as in *The Big Turnip* (Tolstoy, 1982) are good examples. Also a child's own writing is highly predictable because the child has control over the language. Children who are beginning readers often find their first success in reading back a sentence they have dictated to an adult to write down on paper. Older, disabled, or remedial readers also have found success in writing their own booklets on topics that interest them.

A book can also be predictable just because a child has heard it one or more times before. Many adults wearily marvel at the limitless number of times some books are pulled off the shelves. Children listen with such delight and anticipation as if it were the first time the story had been read to them. One of Ryan's favorite books that he read over and over with my assistance is a little known trade book (Zion, 1959) about a boy who earns money "plant sitting" for neighbors who are away on vacation. For an 11-year-old boy with reading disabilities whose family has difficulty making ends meet, this story about earning money, helping one's neighbors, and being an independent problem solver may have satisfied Ryan's fantasy that he would some day be independent and someone whom others depended upon.

It is interesting and sometimes poignantly enlightening to watch which children pick which books. A wonderful but sad story is *I'll Always Love You* (Wilhelm, 1985). It is about a little boy's puppy who grows up and grows old and dies. It is a favorite of many children in my classroom but especially for Alan. Like many children in the room, Alan has experienced many losses in his life. He lost his father to divorce partly as a result of alcoholism and physical abuse. Nevertheless, Alan still worries about his father and sometimes runs away to be with his father and teenage step-brothers. Recently his pet dog died. *I'll Always Love You* seems to help Alan cope with his losses on many levels.

Strategies That Emphasize Meaning

When I am a child's reading partner, I concentrate on modeling important reading strategies that emphasize meaning. For example, a simple strategy to use with beginning readers is for the adult to read along in the story pausing at the end of some sentences to allow the child to supply the predictable ending word or phrase. With more proficient readers, I take turns reading paragraphs or pages with the child. If the child gets stuck on an unknown word, I might chose simply to supply the word to keep the momentum of the story going. At other times, it may be appropriate to help a student use semantic and syntactic clues along with a minimal amount of graphophonic clues (i.e., the beginning letters of a word) to help him or her discover the word. Overemphasizing graphophonic clues is burdensome and inefficient. The most important strategy is to emphasize that the child be involved in getting the author's meaning. I listen to see if the child self-corrects on important miscues that significantly obstruct the meaning of the passage. If the child does not self-correct, I will ask the child to read the sentence again because it did not make sense to me. Teachers can model this strategy when they read to the child so that beginning readers can see that even proficient readers make mistakes but reread and self-correct so that sentences do make sense.

Developing Independence through Choices

Developing independence is an important goal in reading instruction, and allowing students to make choices is a motivational feature that fosters independence. Partners sharing time is only one activity in which students choose their reading materials in my class. A sustained, silent reading period of 15 to 20 minutes is a popular daily activity in which the children may choose one or two books to read by themselves. When children have a turn at the tape recorder with ear phones, they have an array of story cassettes from which to choose, including such favorites as *E.T.* (Spielberg & Magnon, 1982), *Snow White* (Disney, 1970), and *Tikki-Tikki-Tembo* (Mosel, 1971). Science books about animals and space, books about monsters, and joke books are popular when my children visit the school library. Although they seldom have assigned homework, I reinforce their choice to take books home to read.

Even basal readers are used and displayed like trade books in our room, and children have the option of choosing stories from them or checking them out to take home. From time to time, I ask a child to choose a story from a particular basal so that I can check his or her level of proficiency. I also use the basal reading workbooks for this purpose or to cover skills pertaining to comprehension, dictionary usage, and word structure analysis within meaningful contexts. But the main purpose in using the workbooks is to foster sustained independent concentration through focused problem-solving exercises. Special education students too often become quite dependent on a teacher and therefore need encouragement and reinforcement when they are successful at figuring out directions and answers on their own. We are fortunate to have a basal workbook series (Durr *et al.*, 1982) that encourages flexible and independent use. I even allow my students to choose which workbook pages they want to do. The pages are colorful and inviting, with easy-to-understand directions and an emphasis on meaningful stories and paragraphs. There is enough repetition of skills throughout the workbooks that it is only occasionally necessary to assign particular pages for areas that need more practice. If a child is not finding success in one workbook, he or she can choose to work in a different-level workbook. Students do not need to complete all the pages in their workbooks if they are willing and ready to tackle the next higher level.

To find out what reading is about in our room, watch Evelyn, Alan, Tiffany, Ryan, Jerry, and Bob engage in the reading process as they work on reading activities. Do they enjoy listening to and reading books? Can they choose books on their own to either share with a partner or read alone at their desks? Do they check out books to take home? Are they developing appropriate strategies to help them seek out and make sense of an author's meaning? Are they becoming more independent and more confident of their successes in spite of the various levels of proficiency exhibited by their classmates? How do they feel about reading?

ENGAGING CHILDREN IN WRITING: KEEPING A JOURNAL

Academic and Therapeutic Benefits

Like reading, becoming an independent proficient writer is a fundamental language skill in our society. Yet for Evelyn, Alan, Bob, Tiffany, Jerry, and Ryan, writing can be difficult and uncomfortable and possibly even scary for them (see chapter by Parsons). Like reading, it is misleading to say that it is always fun, especially for the student with emotional and language-learning problems. In fact, it may be a more difficult activity than reading for teachers to promote because there are no stacks of colorful, inviting adventures to get lost in as there are in books. The responsibility is on the child to generate the sentences and to take the risk of putting these sentences on paper for others to read.

Regardless of the difficulties, a child's own writing has both academic and therapeutic benefits. Academically, writing can reinforce the reading process, and conversely, reading can enhance the writing process. Both processes involve focusing on and manipulating the semantic, syntactic, and graphophonic systems of the written language. In reading, the child is trying to get the meaning or message of what the author has written. In writing, the child is trying to generate and communicate his or her own thoughts or message to a reader. Although not exactly the same, the two processes complement one another. As in the reading process, modeling and practice can help writing to become an effective, practical, and creative tool of communication.

With my students, I have observed that writing can produce benefits therapeutically as well as academically. Just as reading can help verify and illuminate our inner struggles and fantasies through characters who grapple with similar thoughts and situations, writing can be a way to express and understand our thoughts, wishes, and feelings, first privately and then, perhaps, through sharing them with others so that they can come to know us better. Keeping a daily journal is a simple way for beginning writers to experience the academic and therapeutic benefits of writing.

An Accepting Atmosphere

Although most children come to enjoy the opportunity to keep a daily journal, I find that certain conditions combine together to enhance the environment for journal writing: trust, privacy, modeling, invented spelling when needed, and opportunities for sharing. The very nature of keeping a journal requires a high level of trust between the children and the teacher. My students understand that I am more interested in what they have to write about than in mechanical correctness. I do not correct or mark on their journals. Still, because many children are quite concerned with spelling, I demonstrate strategies to help them feel comfortable with writing if they ask for help.

Spelling is a developmental skill that is often learned as the child experiments with phonetic approximations to the conventional spelling of a word. These approximations are known as "invented spellings." Invented spellings are necessary for beginning spellers not only because it frees them from worries about making mistakes so that they can concentrate on expressing their message but because it helps them to think about words and to generate new knowledge about our written language system (Gentry, 1987).

Children, in time, progress along developmental stages in spelling and make the successful transition from invented spellings to conventional spelling and to a proficient level in using a dictionary. Of course, a child seriously disabled in phonetic processing and visual memory of words will usually have more difficulty with all stages of spelling, including beginning and sophisticated invented spellings, conventional spelling, and an efficient use of a dictionary. I sometimes write a rhyming-patterned word for them on the board when they ask how to spell a certain word so that they may actively and easily experience success. Usually I just ask the child how he or she thinks the word is spelled and write it down as they guess the letters. They are often correct or very close. I have known teachers who work with older students with spelling disabilities who recommend the use of a computer lexicon proofreading program.

Another condition that fosters journal writing is the opportunity to read what they have written to someone if they choose to do so. I am delighted when children enjoy sharing their entries with the class because they learn from and about each other in this way. Additionally, listening to what their classmates have written in their journals helps to provide them with ideas and alternative models of writing.

The children feel free to write about whatever they want. Only rarely have I had to set up certain limitations on what they share with the class. For example, one boy graphically described a dream he had in his journal and then volunteered to read it to the class. The dream was about a girl in our class who was in a house that was blown up, and her body parts were scattered around the world. Sensing my own and other children's strong negative reactions to this, I immediately instituted a policy that the names of people we knew could not be used except with their permission—extending the idea of privacy and respect of other people's feelings.

Some structure and modeling usually help the students to get started with their journal writing. My two basic requirements for writing in a journal are first, that the date be written correctly at the top of the page (which they can copy off the calendar or chalkboard), and second, that they do write something. I have devised a simple five-step chart that I keep posted to aid the students visually. These five steps are (1) date, (2) think, (3) write, (4) illustrate, and (5) share. The last two steps are optional. Step 2, thinking of what to write, is difficult for some children. Because Andrew and I are writing in a journal at the same time that the children are writing, we can model the writing process and share with them that sometimes it is difficult to think of topics. It helps of course if journal writing follows a discussion. Sometimes I circulate among the children commenting on what they have written. If they need ideas about what to write, I ask them questions about what they have been doing or what they are thinking or feeling. I emphasize that I cannot think for them and that it is okay for them to spend a little time thinking about what they want to write. For beginning writers who look like they are stuck, I offer to take dictation from them and have them read it back to me and then copy it into their journals. I help them to appreciate that the thoughts and words are their own and that I merely helped them put their thoughts on paper.

Reading between the Lines

The amount that the children write varies from day to day and varies among children. Sometimes they write a few short sentences, repeating them each day; at other times, they write more colorfully and express more interesting ideas. A major challenge is not to assume that children who write only a few, short repetitive sentences are not expressing something important. Jerry's journal entries are a case in point. He is the youngest and least skillful writer in our class, yet Jerry says a great deal while writing very little. When he first came to the center, he was very quiet and depressed. In his journal he repeatedly wrote, "I am dead" or "I am sad" and would illustrate these entries with a picture of himself in a coffin (see Figure 1).

More recently, for several days in a row, Jerry had written the following three sentences in his journal: "I am happy. I am mad. I am sad." I sat down beside him, read his first sentence out loud, and asked him, "because . . . ?" looking at him and indicating that I wanted him to finish the sentence. He answered, "Because I am." I read aloud his next sentence and asked again, "because . . . ?" and he answered, "Because my brothers ran away from home last night." Once again, after reading his last sentence I asked, "because . . . ?" and he answered, "Because I miss them" (see Figure 2).

With journal entries such as Jerry's, I am given an opportunity to share a private moment with a child who may not have otherwise spoken directly with me about an experience or feeling. In Jerry's case, when his team met during their weekly meeting to share information confidentially, I discovered that Jerry was expressing similar themes and information in his individual therapy time.

Most journal entries are not as revealing as some of Jerry's are. Usually the children write about their friends or their pets or about

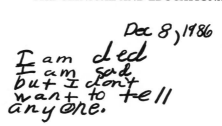

Dec 8, 1986

I am ded
I am sad
but I don't
want to tell
anyone.

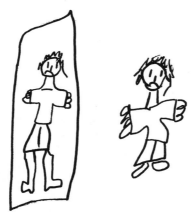

Figure 1.

April 7, 1986

I am happy
because I am.

I am Mad
because my brothers ran away.

I am sad
because I miss my brothers.

Figure 2.

birthdays or holidays or a favorite TV character. Although a child at our center senses in a broader context that the team shares information as a way of helping children and their families, I think the children appreciate that a journal is personal or private writing and that like other aspects of their lives and experiences will be accepted and treated sensitively.

INTEGRATING CREATIVE ACTIVITIES: GOLDEN OPPORTUNITIES

Special Occasions

In addition to books and journals, there are almost limitless language activities that any teacher may use to engage students in reading and writing. Special occasions arise in which students can write thank-you notes to staff members or make birthday cards for parents and therapists or leave notes to the custodian or cook. Special events and themes can be integrated into traditional school units. Literature, science, history, geography, sports, holidays, seasons, and weather are some of the subjects that can come alive when students are involved actively with such themes.

During the early fall of this year, our bulletin boards were full of drawings, maps, news clippings, and hand-written papers that reflected the children's interest in the Olympics taking place in South Korea. I videotaped a few segments such as the exciting diving and swimming competitions. After viewing them, the children became newspaper sports writers describing the events. A further outgrowth came from a chart of the flags of other countries, including South Korea. They found the variety of flags fascinating, and each child enthusiastically designed a colorful flag of his or her own imaginary country. Later in the fall, olympic gold turned to autumn gold as children wrote poetic lists of nature's golden "medals," such as the harvest moon, sunshine, yellow daisies, and juicy apples. Each poem, written neatly on goldenrod paper, received a bright yellow aspen leaf "gold medal" taped to the paper.

November's presidential election and January's inauguration were timely news events that motivated several writing assignments. The children wrote short essays on what problems they would tackle if they were president. Later they conveyed these concerns in serious letters to the new president. On a more humorous note, campaign posters were made for Morris, the cat. We knew he wanted to be the Feline Party's candidate from information on a Morris Calendar that we had in the room.

In October, Columbus Day facts were enlivened with maps and flags of Spain, Italy, and Portugal. At Thanksgiving, we expanded the study of history to include themes of dreams, hardships, friendships with Indians, and freedom of religion. Soon December followed with a study of holiday customs that some of the children celebrated in their homes, such as lighting Chanukah candles, baking cookies, and writing a letter to Santa Claus. New Year's resolutions were written following a discussion about setting goals and making wishes. These included changes we really wanted to make for fun as well as bothersome bad habits that we wanted to break. Jerry's list included a wish to play more hockey and stop fighting with his brother. Ryan's first resolution was to "know something."

Knowing Something

"Knowing something" is important not only for learning-disabled Ryan but for all children's self-esteem as well as their education. Children are pleased when they have the opportunity to learn and demonstrate their newly acquired knowledge. Following the presidential inauguration, the students became interested in some of the presidents and liked to compete in reciting facts and playing trivial-pursuit-type games about the presidents. Such facts included which presidents are pictured on the $20.00 bill, the nickel, or the dime; which presidents were assassinated; and who was president the year they were born.

Knowledge of history, science, and other subjects can be learned in many ways. Children who are not proficient readers often become excellent observers and use the medium of television to learn about the world. Though Bob is not proficient enough to read the newspaper and may not be for a long time, he initiates discussions on current events news that he has seen on television—*Good Morning, America* or *The Today Show*—while he is getting ready for school. We have watched the excellent public television series *Voyage of the Mimi* (1984) and learned to write factual reports about whales and oceans from information gleaned from the televised programs. A film shown on Martin Luther King, Jr.'s birthday introduced new words and concepts such as *prejudice, nonviolence, boycott,* and *brotherhood.* The children first discussed and then wrote about their feelings and opinions of what they saw on the film. Later they wrote factual biographies or reports about the events in Martin Luther King, Jr.'s life. Understanding the difference between fact and opinion helps children not only to write more appropriate reports but assists them in sorting out feelings from factual events. This process has generalized to other areas of their lives and has helped them in their discussions of peer problems that arise on the playground or bus.

Innovative Book Presentations

Presenting information in a variety of ways can be motivating to students and teachers as an enjoyable departure from the daily routine. The students at our center always enjoy watching *Reading Rainbow* (1984), another excellent public television series relating good books to background information in science and the social studies fields. Each televised program concludes with a segment of short, snappy book reviews by children in order to encourage the viewing audience to choose these books to enjoy on their own.

Last year I asked my students to write a brief summary about a favorite book that they wanted to persuade the others to read that departed from the usual way of reviewing books. Dean, who enjoyed the status of class clown, had come to the front of the classroom to share his summary. He hopped up on his desk and, mimicking the style of the televised *Reading Rainbow* book reviews, gave an enthusiastic summary of his book. We clapped at Dean's performance, and the other students followed his theatrical lead. I asked them if they would like to make a videotape of their book reviews. All the children were excited about the idea, but when our audiovisual specialist came a few days later, I discovered that Matt, a shy self-conscious 12-year-old, did not want to see himself on tape. After some negotiations, Matt was happy to be safely in the background as the "director."

There were embarrassed giggles as the children viewed the tape, but it was obvious that they were pleased by their performances. We decided to make invitations and refreshments and invite the other three classes to view our production. The *Reading Rainbow* teacher's guide (1984) provided us with a recipe for rainbow-colored cookies, and the children prepared brightly decorated programs.

Encouraging Creative Fantasy

Purely creative writing assignments can be a fun way to practice writing skills and can also give an opportunity for expressing feelings and fears. For Halloween, my students wrote either a real or imagined scary story (usually a mixture of both), and these stories were read by the eerie light of the jack-o-lantern's candle. Another time, the children wrote imaginary humorous stories from a pet's point of view. This assignment was very motivating because we had just heard *Bunnicula* (Howe & Howe, 1979), a humorous story about a new pet bunny who upsets the lives of the other household pets and family members. Children who did not have a pet had an opportunity to imagine one in their home. All types of literature can become models for student writing. Following a unit on fairy tales, Alan wrote the following short fairy tale that closely parallels some of the conflict he has seen in his own life.

The title—A Queen and King

One day a queen kicked the king out of the house. And the king sade HELP and he landed in a dragens hole. And burnt his but and he got his burnt but out of there.

Play Acting

Themes from literature and television and real-life adventures are often woven into the fabric of the children's play as well as into their writing. Often they play-act during their recess and free play activities, reenacting scenes from books or television programs or from real life, or by making up their own stories spontaneously on the playground or in the classroom. One cold wintery day when the children were indoors for recess, Tiffany, Evelyn, and Alan spontaneously developed a play about a queen, a princess, and a burglar. They made simple costumes and props from construction paper and cardboard as the story evolved. I did not even realize they were acting out a play because I was talking in the hall with Jerry, who had just entered our program a few weeks before. He had been very disruptive and was having difficulty taking a time-out to settle himself down. Jerry's attention was suddenly drawn to the actors; he looked longingly in their direction. "Too bad," I mused, "that you are missing out on all the fun. Perhaps you would like to be in the play, too." He quickly completed his time-out calmly, then asked the children if he could be in their play. He was assigned the part of the queen's servant, meekly (and willingly) fetching things for her. They made up the story as they went along, speaking with animation to one another—giving directions and following directions. Evelyn was the beautiful and timid princess; Tiffany was the haughty and bossy queen; and Alan was the mean, threatening burglar. Queen Tiffany used her magical powers to turn Alan, the bad burglar, into a frog and then into "a good man who knew how to behave."

I congratulated them on the play and suggested to them that the younger children's class might enjoy seeing them perform it later that same afternoon. They were delighted by the idea and sent a messenger (Servant Jerry) next door to deliver a written invitation. At the end of the performance, in keeping with their earlier spontaneity, the queen and the princess circulated around the audience tapping each child with their cardboard wands and asked each to state a wish. Bob, an angry and oppositional boy, poignantly said as he was tapped, "I wish somebody would love me."

Feelings and wishes, reading and writing, work and play—all are integrated into the daily events of the six children who share a therapeutic classroom with Andrew and me.

REFERENCES

Charlip, R. (1964). *Fortunately.* New York: Parents' Magazine Press.

Disney, W. (1970). *Snow White and the seven dwarfs.* (Cassette Recording No. RA9). Burbank, CA: Walt Disney Educational Media Co.

Durr, W. K., LePere, J. M., Pikulski, J. J., & Shaw, S. (Eds.). (1982). *Sunshine.* Boston: Houghton Mifflin Co.

Gentry, J. R. (1987). *Spel . . . is a four-letter word.* Portsmouth, NH: Heinemann Educational Books.

Howe, D., & Howe, J. (1979). *Bunnicula.* New York: Avon Books.

Mosel, A. (1971). *Tikki-Tikki-Tembo.* (Cassette Recording No. 0590-60690-5). New York: Scholastic.

Parnell, D. (1987a). *The little red hen.* Lewiston, ME: Ladybird Books.

Parnell, D. (1987b). *The ugly duckling.* Lewiston, ME: Ladybird Books.

Reading rainbow: A guide for teachers. (1984). Lincoln, NE: Great Plains National Instructional Television Library.

Rhodes, L. K. (1981). I can read! Predictable books as resources for reading and writing instruction. *Reading Teacher, 34,* 511–518.

Sperry, A. (1940). *Call it courage.* New York: Macmillan.

Spielberg, S., & Magon, J. (Producers). (1982). *E.T., the extra-terrestrial.* (Cassette Recording No. 1560C). Burbank, CA: Buena Vista Records.

Tolstoy, A. (1982). *The big turnip.* In W. K. Durr, J. M. LePere, J. J. Pikulski, & S. Shaw (Eds.), *Sunshine.* Boston: Houghton Mifflin Co.

Voyage of the Mimi. (1984). New York: The Bank Street College of Education.

White, E. B. (1952). *Charlotte's web.* New York: Harper & Row.

Wilhelm, H. (1985). *I'll always love you.* New York: Crown Publishers.

Zion, G. (1959). *The plant sitter.* New York: Harper & Brothers.

7

Behind the Bottom Line

A Cautionary Tale for New Teachers of Troubled and Troublesome Children

PHYLLIS C. PARSONS

INTRODUCTION

> For reasons we couldn't define
> The young teacher wouldn't resign.
> In spite of her schooling
> She said, "I'm not fooling,
> This can't be the whole bottom line."

The education teachers receive is the bottom line when they walk into any classroom with their name on the door, but when working with emotionally disturbed youngsters, the teachers who survive have learned how to seek, find, and use what lies behind the bottom line (Cohen, 1966).

Children, in general, have a way of making you feel, as a new teacher, that your preparation for teaching has little to do with the real world. This feeling is magnified when working with emotionally disturbed children. Lessons that are designed to motivate children, to maintain their interest, or to stimulate individual and group thinking may be effective in a group of 30 children in regular schools; they are likely to go nowhere in the classroom of six children in a day treatment center. Management techniques that were relatively successful in a regular classroom

---

PHYLLIS C. PARSONS • The Day Care Center, Department of Psychiatry, University of Colorado Health Sciences Center, Denver, Colorado 80262.

have as much impact as a pebble tossed in a lake. The new teacher, if he or she has time to reflect, wonders: Can group discussions, creative art and writing, field trips, and a host of other seemingly exciting activities ever be used with emotionally disturbed children? Can the teacher ever get beyond containment?

The qualities common to teachers who are effective with normal children must be tuned many times finer in those who work with emotionally disturbed children. You will be tested and tested and then tested again before these children trust you enough to explore their world within the structure you provide. Having a sense of humor, a strong sense of self, and a great deal of patience, each takes on a new depth of meaning when you discover that it will take a very long time before these children will trust you enough to follow you down the learning road.

What appears to be a paradoxical approach to behavior management soon becomes a rule of thumb. The term *rigid flexibility* is an example that comes to mind. This approach involves the use of such invaluable abstract tools of your trade as timing, pacing, and being ready to substitute alternate plans at the very last minute within a firmly structured environment. In effect, you need to learn to be skilled in determining when to introduce an activity, how much time to give it, and how to move away from it and into another activity smoothly albeit suddenly (Kounin, 1970). If you are able to apply "rigid flexibility," you are more likely to enjoy the challenges presented in this area of special education.

In addition to working with children, you will be expected to relate to the children's parents and to other staff members who are trained in other disciplines. You will develop and sharpen your sensitivity to anticipate and "read," not only where the children are coming from, but also, where they are going. You will learn these things slowly, and most of them will be taught by the children you teach. Your supervisor can offer a different perspective, problem-solve situations with you, and help you to become aware of changes in yourself. Above all, a supervisor can listen. However, a supervisor cannot tell you what to do, give you a list of "if–then" equations, or tell you what will work and what will not; the supervisor does not know. What works for one teacher and child may not work for another. There are no recipes. When teaching emotionally disturbed children in a treatment center or in a mainstreamed school, the most you can start with is that the only thing predictable is unpredictability.

Therefore, whether you enter the arena freshly certified with diploma in hand or by way of experience in a regular classroom, you are going to learn more about yourself, kids, and teaching than you dream-ed existed if you choose. However, if you have a rigid inflexibility and cannot adapt, forget the postgraduate course behind the bottom line and select another profession.

ERRORS

Taking chances when you are working in a goldfish bowl is a risky business. It is embarrassing, to say the least, to make mistakes in front of your peers, but this happens in a treatment center. It is lunch time and Jim's ninth birthday. Jim's psychotherapist stops by to say, "Happy Birthday." Jim's been "hyper" all morning, and his behavior worsens at the lunch table. The therapist tries to calm him and settle him down. Jim yells and tips over his chair. This behavior quickly ripples to others (Kounin, 1970). Another minute, and chaos reigns. You intervene by removing a "cussing" Jim and his lunch to the hall where he stays until the lunch period ends. Later, the team and therapist suggest that the intervention could have been handled more constructively at the lunchroom table with teacher and therapist labeling and working on the birthday behavior. An error? It does not really matter. Sure there were alternatives. To you the priority was to prevent the ripple from becoming a wave. You made a judgment call. You will have to make them everyday. Some will be good calls, others you will wish you could recall, but you have to take risks. The important thing is to do something. Errors of commission can be worked through, but errors of omission are often destructive and are to be avoided.

TARGETS

Ordinarily we know when we set ourselves up to be a target, but the teacher of disturbed children is always a target. At a day treatment center, youngsters bring their home hassles to school. Very often the first time you have to make a normal demand on a youngster loaded with home tensions you get the barrage. And the dose may be large. You get what belongs to a parent, possibly a sibling, or other caregiver. Sometimes the behavior can be labeled for the child with varying degrees of success. The important aspect in this onslaught is to recognize that you are the nearest and safest target. If you take arrows personally, you only set the stage for power struggles and control battles that inevitably result in no-win, anxiety-provoking situations. Remember, too, the target has two sides, and at times you may be the one dragging personal baggage into the classroom. For example, did you have a sleepless night, a fight with a friend or spouse, or is there a serious illness or death in your family? Assuming you are aware of your feelings, it behooves you to control them unless you truly need to be a masochist.

TALK! TALK! TALK!

Most teachers talk too much (Haring & Phillips, 1962). The more you talk, the more opportunity you give your group to practice tuning out. Remember, many of these kids have a short attention span. A teacher talks to get a point across. To make sure the kids understand, the teacher says the same thing a half dozen times. Worse than that, however, is the way teachers tend to treat kids who answer a question. Consider this dialogue:

Teacher: Who can tell us four ways of receiving information? Jill, can you tell us four ways we get information?

Jill: We read the newspaper, and talk, and listen to the radio and watch TV.

Teacher: Good. We read newspapers, we talk, we listen to the radio and we watch and listen to the television. Are there other ways we get information besides the radio, television, newspapers, and talking, as Jill told us?

A bit redundant, perhaps? You laugh, but teachers are known to do this, even in regular schools. Jill must wonder if she said it right the first time. Why do teachers parrot children's responses, as well as their own? Why? To make sure everyone hears and understands, of course. Think back to your own classroom days. These are the repetitions you began to tune out until at times you tuned out the important things, too.

Another example of teacher overtalk occurs because we want so much to spare these youngsters some of the painful childhood experiences we suffered through, that we fall into the trap of, "When I was young like you, I . . . ," and we talk, but they do not necessarily hear. To them, we are teachers, and as far as they are concerned, teachers were never children. Besides, each individual has to grow through his or her own experiences.

Such excess talk fosters less listening. One of the teachers at the Day Care Center many years ago advised his trainees to apply the OLI (rhymes with Polly) principle to their teaching. OLI translates into Observe, Listen, Inquire. When we decrease our talk, it is surprising how much the children tell us, as well as how much we can hear what they are not saying.

HUMOR

Norman Cousins (1979), whose life was at risk, attributed the restoration of his health to humor. As I mentioned before, a healthy sense of humor is essential for teachers, too. When you are able to see the funny side of a situation and can laugh at yourself, you are on the right track to extending your own life. There are other advantages as well. Your colleagues will enjoy working with you; the children will seek you out; you will begin to realize that you are enjoying your work. Strangely enough, humor, in its broad meaning, is alien to most troubled children. They seldom laugh when they are having fun, perhaps because they do not trust the good feelings they are experiencing. They will laugh a hostile kind of laugh, however, at another's misfortune. The following examples illustrate my point:

> Ginny was learning to roller skate and took very frequent falls. Each fall was punctuated with sideline laughter.

> Harry wore his new birthday western shirt to school. No one said much about it until he spilled model airplane paint all over the sleeve, then everyone laughed.

> Sylvia's ceramic pony was beautiful when it came out of the kiln, but no one paid attention to it. She dropped it, however, and the laughter came as it lay in pieces on the floor.

Every day there are many opportunities to help these children to distinguish between what is *hurtful* humor and what is *healthy* humor. One very powerful way to learn this distinction is to practice and model it yourself (Keelan, 1987).

SURPRISES

The cockroach's survival over thousands of centuries is attributed to its adaptive capabilities. Most children who are emotionally handicapped display little ability to "roll with the punches" or "go with the flow," even in their classrooms, which often provide the most stable, predictable island in their daily lives. A foolproof way, for example, to guarantee a chaotic day is to rearrange the furniture in the classroom without discussing it with the children, even when the reasons for doing so are sound ones. It had occurred to you that Jennie needed to be moved further away from Tess, and Lyle's team had suggested that because he has finally begun to relate to a peer, now is the time to seat him next to Vern. You have also noticed that the typewriter is being misused, and you decided to move it to a safer, more visible location. From mind to motion, the changes are effected in a matter of minutes at the end of the day after the children have left. And, as a last-minute thoughtful touch, you check that the name labels on the desks are intact so that the children will not have any difficulty in finding their desks in the new location.

Now let us move to the following morning where we will see a slightly modified reenactment of the story of the *Three Bears*, when they return from their walk to find their home in an altered state. But in our scenario, the bears are the children. Most people, including children, will automatically move to the familiar; they are not likely to look for their name labels first. No sooner do they realize that the room is not how they had left it the day before when the looks of confusion on their faces turn to looks of anger and distrust. One child breaks the silence: "Who put their stuff in my desk?" This question does not wait for an answer but is followed immediately by action: the dumping of the desk's contents on the floor. Another child asks, "How come my desk got over here?" And then there is a scurry of activity when they each begin to relocate the desks to their old positions. Then comes the last question: "Who's been messing around in our room?" You get the flavor of the depth of feelings being expressed. What do you do? You could be cowardly and blame it on the custodian, or more appropriately, take responsibility (modeling the expected behavior) and acknowledge that you did it, explain all the reasons for so doing, and turn the incident into a learning situation, involving the children in the discussion.

Discussing the changes with the children individually and as a group in advance—what is referred to in the education jargon as prealerting (Kounin, 1970) is sound therapeutic teaching practice. It will avoid a lot of the anger, anxiety, and mistrust that is bound to erupt when the children meet unexpected changes. Furniture changes are but one of many surprises to avoid whenever possible. Schedule changes, field trips, observers, and your own absence, if possible, are other changes that should trigger in your mind the word *prealert*.

Perhaps as you are reading this you are thinking that I am too concerned about protecting the children (or myself) and that the situation that evolves is a piece of reality that provides the opportunity for dealing with legitimate emotions. That may be true, and you hope you have done your best to capitalize on the positive aspects of this situation. It is my belief, however, that there is a sufficient number of events for which you cannot prealert the children. To drive my point home, it may be helpful for you to put yourself in the following circumstances:

Remember how disappointed, angry, and upset you got when the rain poured down from leaden skies and you knew your plans were doomed? You kitchen counter was covered with fried chicken, and all the other picnic necessities were readied with no place to go. How quickly were you able to bring to bear your well-honed adaptive skills? Or remember when you signed in for your doctor's appointment and were told you would have to reschedule because the doctor was dealing with an emergency and would not be able to see you? Compare these situations to when the child's therapist calls the last minute, after the last minute, or possibly not at all, to cancel the appointment because of an emergency. Your adaptive capacities surely far exceed those of these children, so avoid surprises, and, whenever possible, prealert.

RIGHTING WRITING WRONGS

Probably more power struggles occur over writing than any other aspect of the school program. Writing is important, writing legibly is more important, and writing legibly with meaning is the ultimate goal. Unfortunately, even endless searches behind the bottom line reveal no magical quick fix to these needed communication skills. We know some of the causes of resistance, but the cures are far less clear.

Examples of the obstacles to writing include perceptual problems, poor fine-motor coordination, lack of models who write, behavioral problems, fear of risking criticism, embarrassment about one's poor handwriting skills, and a reluctance at exposing one's ideas. Many children who resist writing will tell you that it is hard and it is dumb. Translated, these statements usually mean that they have had a few successful writing experiences in their previous school; their papers have been "red penciled," and they have spent long and arduous periods writing the material over and over again. Sometimes the mistakes are shown to others, especially to parents, as evidence of their poor performance, and frequently this has resulted in punishment. They learn early, therefore, that their writing openly exposes too much of themselves to potential criticism and reprimand. In other words, it is an activity that is closely associated with shame and failure and is, therefore, highly emotionally charged. Types of remedies attempted depend on the age of the child and the child's specific writing ability. The initial goal of the teacher is desensitization (Blom, Rudnick, & Weiman, 1966). I have found that this is best achieved by scheduling frequent doses of writing every day in many different contexts. Grades are never given; red pencil marks are taboo. Gradually, however, pupil and teacher expectations converge, especially when the writing tasks they are asked to do are based on realistic objectives.

Dosing and pacing are two keys to desensitizing writing traumata.

The specific activities you select for dosing and pacing depend on the children's ages and their level of writing ability. For those who are more proficient writers, taking one or more sentences down from dictation every day at the same time of day has worked well. These children learn to correct their own papers from a model I write on the blackboard for them to see. However, for those children who are unable to write independently, I select appropriate material for each of them to copy, and I provide immediate feedback to them when they have finished their tasks.

As a general rule, you should assign only parts of long workbook pages, give choices to the children, challenge their strengths, and also make allowances for their fears. Accept writing on an erasable slate or chalkboard to make corrections easier and mistakes less humiliating. You will find that down the line, your expectations for them and their expectations for themselves will begin to converge.

Coming up with relatively successful activities and strategies to continue to stimulate the writing habit is not without its problems. In addition to relying on your own understanding of the individual child's learning style and your own pool of curriculum ideas and resources, you may want to find out what the other teachers at the center are finding successful with their groups of children. Activities geared for younger or older children than the ones you are working with can frequently be adapted to meet your children's needs as well (see the chapter by Carol Lee).

When evaluating the children's written work, be honest as well as constructive with them. In most cases, they are very aware of the quality of their own productions and will be more willing to trust your word in other situations if they have found you an honest, nonpunitive evaluator in this one. This problem is especially heightened at the time of your report card conference with parents. It is important to prealert the children to the fact that you will show a specified group of papers to their parents at your meeting with them but that they may take out one of them if they wish. Similarly, you should ask the child for permission before displaying his or her work in the classroom. Both of these acts of respect on your part may help to give the children some experience with the opportunity to control some elements of their own lives, possibly for the first time ever.

HAPPY HOLIDAYS

Never in my training as a special education teacher was I taught that for most disturbed children vacations are unwanted and holidays are "traumadays." Until thrust into the middle of the shrieking crescendo of anxiety, we assume that Halloween, Chanukah, Christmas, and Valentine's Day, for example, are basically times for fun. As with most people in the real world, many of these holidays are perceived with a modicum of ambivalence to outright paralyzing anxiety. In spite of this, we assume that children look forward to vacations as much as we do. Definitely not so, and, as teachers, we are likely to pay dearly for every school holiday and vacation. (Of course, the parents of these children have also expressed similar concerns.)

Halloween

Halloween, with its ghosts and ghouls and haunted houses, stimulates already overactive imaginations. In addition, most costumes do little for poor self-images, especially when met by such purposefully disparaging remarks by their friends as "What a dumb thing to wear"; "You wore the same thing last year"; or "You dressed like a girl because you act like one, anyway." Even the children who elect to forego the costume are subject to such barbs as "Poor sport!"; "Oh, I thought that was your costume"; or "You wear that same mask every day!"

Although it is neither desirable nor possible to dispel all the excitement and anxieties stirred up by Halloween, it is possible to engage in more neutral activities. These might include making a 3-D scarecrow, planning party games, drawing faces on pumpkins with magic markers, baking Halloween cookies, or completing a prestarted Halloween picture. A high degree of structure also will reduce the volatile potential of this holiday.

The Long Winter Vacation

Christmas and Chanukah, with their accompanying winter break time that we, as teachers, look forward to, is not an easy time for these youngsters. Where we see this midwinter holiday as an opportunity to refresh ourselves, to have fun, and to be with loved ones, many of these children have a very different response. For them, this holiday is closely associated with unfulfilled dreams and wishes. For example, those who have experienced abandonment by one or both biological parents may be consumed by the wish to be reunited with them; no other gift will satisfy these youngsters. On the other hand, some may be shifted between parents living in different parts of the country and have to be confronted by the renewal of old family battles and frustrating attempts at reestablishing close relationships that are continually weakened by long absences.

Then there may be the concern that they will not receive any gifts because they are so bad and, in turn, they behave badly in order to prove that they are right. In addition, the prospect of spending many lonely days at home without friends, structure, and discipline is a dismal one, indeed. In effect, the staff at the center may give the children holiday parties and holiday gifts, but they also take away from them a consistent, caring, and highly predictable 2 weeks.

Valentine's Day

Probably the most difficult of the traumadays is Valentine's Day. Hearts begin appearing by the end of January, and, before the groundhog determines the season's changes, anxiety begins its heartfelt rise. Most of the year, through fighting, running, and blaming others, they manage to mask these fears and the dearth of caring relationships. In fact, these maladaptive attempts to "cover up" are likely to get louder and more intense just before Valentine's Day, ensuring that they have, indeed, made themselves totally unlovable, the return of the self-fulfilling prophecy. In truth, these children seldom see themselves as lovable and worthy of friends, and, in fact, most have experienced very little acceptance by adults and peers alike. Thus Valentine messages become cruel symbols of rejection and loss. The number of Valentine cards they receive, therefore, provides them with a concrete measure of their worst fears. Paradoxically, those who receive a lot of Valentine cards may be unable to accept them because, no matter what, they continue to feel unworthy; and those who get only a few are deeply hurt because they have the proof of their worthlessness. This is known in the classical literature as a "no-win situation."

Many of these children are afraid to give these symbols of "I love you" or "I like you" because they may not get any back. More cards are forgotten at home or in the car than seems possible by chance alone, and the wastebasket ends up being the biggest recipient either way. The teacher who survives unscathed by the trauma of Valentine's Day with a group of troubled youngsters, deserves at least one giant Valentine's card for sure!

Holiday and Vacation Remedies

It is no wonder that holidays and long vacations are viewed with apprehension and distaste. On the other hand, you cannot avoid holidays and vacations and you do not really want to; they are a fact of life. Then, what can be done to reduce the high personal costs incurred by these traumadays? First of all, do not get caught up in the festivities too soon and do not prolong the celebrations. Do provide a rockbound structure and deal with the anxious, disruptive behaviors honestly and matter of factly. In other words, show that you understand the feelings and the cause of the negative behaviors but make it clear that you neither encourage nor condone the maladaptive behaviors used to deal with these feelings. This can be done by labeling the feelings, by setting clear limits, and by encouraging the children to substitute adaptive solutions (Blom & Parsons, 1976). Above all, remember that these days, too, shall pass.

TRIP TIPS

Actually, I was told about the value of field trips as an enrichment activity in my teacher training classes. In broad textbook terms, I remembered that a field trip could be an excellent introduction to a study unit, an expansion of a study unit, and/or an excellent culminating activity to a study unit. In addition, though incidentally, it was a good way for children to practice appropriate social skills in public places. The three specific points that stuck with me regarding any excursion off the school premises were (a) that I must obtain a signed permission slip from the parents of every child who passes through the doors of the "big yellow bus"; (b) that every field trip must have a valid purpose in connection with a study unit; and (c) that each child should be aware of this purpose and have a paper to refer to during the trip with the questions on it for which he or she is seeking the answers. As with the training of many professionals working with people, however, some of the details are left to practicum experiences, and so it is with teachers. Thus if field trips are not part of the curriculum activities of the master teachers to whom you are assigned and if you should decide to include them in your curriculum activities, you are going to have to learn through trial and error. In the cautionary tale I relate next, this is what happened to me.

Very early in my career as a special teacher, I decided that as a culminating activity to a study unit on wild animals, my group would make a trip to our local city zoo. This was the first excursion we had ever taken together as a group away from our classroom. As a first step, I decided to make a scouting trip in advance, just to make sure of the exact location of the animals and exhibits I wanted my group to see and to come up with a hand-drawn map of these locations that I would duplicate and give to each child. While carrying out my intent, I saw a big yellow schoolbus pull up at the unloading zone. Doors opened, and one by one, off stepped a line of approximately thirty 8- to 9-year-olds. They gathered around a single tall figure, who suddenly clapped her hands twice. Immediately, the children paired up and waited for the next instructions. The teacher held up a sheaf of papers, and two youngsters came forward, took the papers, and methodically passed them out to their calmly waiting classmates. All at once the teacher pointed decisively at a small person in a blue shirt. As if on command, the blue shirt moved to the teacher's side without comment, bowed its head as the teacher apparently voiced disapproval over something I had missed. Then, as one body, the group moved toward the iron grid fence behind which the tigers paced midst a jungle setting. I left breathing easier, believing that the chapter in my college text on enrichment activities in which field trips were briefly mentioned would work. Worries over next Monday's field trip with a group of seven 8- to 11-year-old emotionally disturbed children were laid to rest.

Monday arrived, and it was not raining; a good omen, I thought. When I arrived at the treatment center, the note in my box informed me that Smitty would be driving the van and would be helping me with the class. Thinking back to the big yellow schoolbus, I felt tempted to say I did not need help, but something told me to keep my mouth shut. The children liked Smitty; he was good with them—firm, soft-spoken, and consistent.

Gathering my precious maps, I was headed for a before-school team meeting when the center secretary called me to report that Mrs. Woods had phoned to tell me that Molly had refused to come to school because she was afraid of the snakes at the zoo, and, therefore, Molly would be left at the baby-sitter's for the day. I sighed fatalistically and continued on to the team meeting. Unfortunately, it ran overtime as we tried to arrange a common time for all to be present for Selby's review conference. Rushing to my classroom, I could see and hear that all was not well:

Jason was poised and ready to land a blow on Barney, who was loudly challenging Jason's ancestry. My intervention was effective in deflecting the blow but too late to dispel angry feelings. Lyle waved a note from his mother in my face while I repeatedly ordered everyone to sit down. The note was not reassuring; Lyle had diarrhea over the weekend and would need access to a bathroom on a minute's notice. I reassured him that there were several toilets on the route to the zoo and that we would find out where the toilets were located immediately on arrival there. (I had neglected to locate them on my hand-drawn maps.) Ella, in excited and anxious tones, told me she'd been sent to her aunt's house for the weekend because her Mom and her mom's boyfriend had gone camping in the mountains. They hadn't returned yet. She did not want to go on the field trip because she might miss the phone call from her aunt that her mother had returned home safely. I told her I didn't want her to miss the trip to the zoo and that we would call from the zoo to find out if a message had been left for her. (I hadn't located the phones at the zoo on my hand-drawn maps.) Selby and Andy were arguing about who was going to sit in the front seat of the van and turned their anger toward me when I drew the seating arrangement on the board, giving them no further choice in the matter.

The atmosphere in the classroom still felt very unsettled by the time Smitty announced at the door that the van was waiting. Together we herded the children into their designated seats. Lyle, green complexioned, panicked 5 minutes into the drive to the zoo so we stopped at the first service station along the route. Several times during the 15-minute drive to the zoo, Andy and Selby and Barney and Lyle managed to reignite their earlier battles. In desperation, I threatened to turn around and come back to school. But each threat prompted cries of, "We'll settle down; we promise!" Meanwhile, Ella sat wringing her hands, asking every minute if we could stop along the way to phone.

Dragging out the details of things that did not go well with this culminating activity would only prolong the pain. Suffice it to say that the only pairings were fighting ones and those between Lyle and the toilet and Ella and the telephone. The maps were used primarily for paper airplanes. There was more interest in the lawn-mowing machines than in the animals. To my extreme embarrassment, several of the children managed to enlist the irate attention of a security guard when they spit chewing gum into the seals' moat, and when we thought we had lost Selby and Barney who, heedless to our commands, chased some roaming banty roosters across the grounds. Threats ranging from loss of free time to no more trips forever fell on deaf ears. After extraordinary efforts by Smitty and me, we managed to get all six children back on the van for the return trip to the center. I began wondering if the scenes of 30 children on the big yellow school bus were simply a figment of my imagination.

Everyone was indescribably relieved to get back to the confines of the classroom. Lyle was only 15 steps from a bathroom; Ella did not hear of her mother's return until just before dismissal time but was within close range of the telephone; and each of the four fighters was placed in one of the four corners of the room.

This first field trip disaster remains among the top 10 most discouraging and devastating experiences of my 20 years of teaching troubled children. At the end of that memorable day, when I was free to reflect on my incompetence with Smitty, I was ready to leave teaching behind me forever. It was Smitty's sense of humor that helped me to resurrect both my sense of humor and my self-confidence. Smitty laughed as we talked about what had happened and said, softly, "How about trying this again tomorrow? It's never as bad the second time around, and this time I'll bring along the leashes and the muzzles." Well, I did not want to try it again tomorrow but maybe at some later date. But more important, I could see the humor in what had happened, and I knew what I would do differently the next time.

Experience is a good but often harsh teacher. You, too, will have plenty of opportunities to learn from that same teacher. However, because this is a collection of cautionary tales, I hope that you will benefit from mine; forewarned is forearmed, and so here are some "trip tips" that you may find helpful:

1. Plan field trips on days other than Monday when the kids need the predictable classroom structure after the weekend.
2. Avoid unnecessary hassles and anxiety by being in the classroom before the children arrive.
3. Make a scouting expedition and be atuned to the location of all of the important places, toilets and telephones included.
4. Plan and rehearse the trip with your group, step by step. Maps and question papers should be familiar to the group before the trip.
5. Take care of the mechanics. Include other adults to help contain the children and let the children and their parents know who these adults will be, what other arrangements have been made, what will be seen, and the rules and expectations for the trip. This process of prealerting should be done several times before the actual trip.
6. Accept help and use other staff who are willing to help. Do not feel embarrassed that there are two or three adults for six or seven children. Just remember, you multiply every disturbed child by 5 and that is the realistic number you are dealing with.
7. Keep the time of the excursion short and to the point.
8. Never make managerial statements (commonly called threats), on which you cannot or are unwilling to follow through. The kids will continue to test you if you do not say what you mean and mean what you say. Your consistency, in effect, makes it safer for them.
9. Finally, expect the unexpected to happen and practice all the things that I referred to earlier: rigid flexibility and laughing at

yourself or at the situation (Keelan, 1987). If you get uptight, the kids will get even more so. They are the barometer of how you are reacting and behaving.

CONSIDER THE PARENTS

When things go wrong, it is human nature to look for someone or something to blame. Changes in routine, the new child who enters the class, a carefully planned lesson that flops, or not feeling well are only a few instances that can result in a bad day, causing you to question your capabilities as a teacher. Often the safest targets for our frustrations are the children's parents. Too quickly we rationalize that a troublesome child would not even be in a treatment center if parents had done their job. Regardless of the enormity of the situation, blame only shifts the problem from the blamer to someone or something else, and there it festers with little hope of resolution.

Instead, consider the parents who live with the troubled and troublesome child. If you feel lousy after a hectic teaching day, how do you suppose the parents feel after years of struggling? You can close the door and get away, but parents do not have that luxury. Imagine yourself in their place for an evening, a weekend, a summer vacation! Every day they have made mistakes just like everyone else. Parents are people, too, with wants, needs, and vulnerabilities similar to yours.

The treatment team meeting is the first place you can begin to develop an understanding of the parents, whom you will eventually meet at parent conferences, family nights, and when they come to the center for their own meetings. Usually they want to help themselves, their child, and you. How can you work with them? Assume a nonjudgmental and nonpatronizing stance; be honest, fair, and tactful; spend more time listening then talking; and phone them periodically with positive rather than negative feedback. Blame creates distance. Learning to understand is a roadway to mutual problem solving.

PROBABLE AND POSSIBLE PROBLEMS

As you must remember to prealert the children to program changes, I am trying to prealert you to situations and events that undoubtedly will confront you early in your teaching. You will develop your own teaching and coping styles, but the more aware you are of the little things that will occur, the more comfortable you will be in dealing with them when they arise.

Personal Possessions

Children bring things from home to school for a variety of reasons. For example, some children may need to "show off" in order to gain attention, acceptance, and, at times, prestige from the other children and/or teacher. Other children may need these objects from home to help them make the transition from home to school. Whatever the reasons, these "things" are likely to cause problems. They get lost, broken, misplaced, or stolen; they cause jealousy, fights, and inattentiveness. Keeping faith with your goal of rigid flexibility, you need to have a policy about bringing personal possessions to school that includes what items are allowed and disallowed; what must stay with you, the teacher, for designated times; and what happens to the items when they fail to serve a constructive purpose such as being attentive to work and getting along with the other children. If there are any doubts as to what items are okay, you are the final arbiter. In other words, nothing is to be brought to school that is not checked through you first. Parents need to know this, too, so that you can work together.

When to Intervene

At first you may feel like making believe that what you just saw did not really happen, or you may feel that by ignoring what you just saw, it will not happen again. Being a just and wise observer and letting things happen naturally also may be supported by your belief that youngsters at a treatment center need to be given the opportunity to work through their problems in a safe environment and that not all fires are damaging. On the other hand, it is unlikely that noxious behavior will stop by ignoring it. In addition to being part of the "testing" of the teacher's ability to provide a safe environment, the behavior may be so ingrained in the child that it is necessary to practice other behaviors in order to increase the frequency of adaptive response patterns. How, then, do you decide which behaviors are harmless and which must be attended to immediately? Which will cause a "ripple effect" (infect the other children) and which will be confined to the child or children directly involved? Which of the harmful behaviors requires what kind and what degree of intervention? And which ones have your top priority when several harmful behaviors are occurring simultaneously (Kounin, 1970)? Obviously, children need to be protected from physical and psychological harm so that they can feel safe. Other situations are less blatant. Your hypervigilance at first will be followed by a knowing vigilance based on your knowledge of each child's background and his or her way of responding. In addition to knowing each child well, however, it is essential that you have, on hand, a wide repertoire of constructive interventions (Long & Newman, 1971) to use at all times, but that gets into how to intervene, a topic for another chapter.

THE CHANGING AND CHALLENGING MILIEU AND YOU

The Milieu

As a member of a multidisciplinary team working in a treatment milieu, you will find yourself dealing with changes continually. Team meetings and scheduled staffings will have to be shifted periodically. You will be asked to host observers who may be visiting the center for a short time. A teacher's absence will find your having to take more children into your classroom or give up your work period to cover someone else's group. Emergency situations involving a former student or one in a transition placement may result in a hastily called meeting away from your class. If you cannot be flexible enough to accept these interruptions in your routine, you will be uptight most of the time, with the staff as well as with the children. Remember what I said earlier? Your group will be the barometer of your psychological state. Sometimes their problems are your problems, and you need to be alert to when that situation exists.

Baubles and Body Parts

The simple message here is that if you have got it, do not flaunt it. These children are easily distracted and sexually stimulated. Channeling their energies into growth-promoting activities can be made more complicated if you inadvertently become the focus of their curiosity and imagination. No, you do not have to present as Grant Wood's "American Gothic" image but be aware that the child who is rolling around on the floor may be looking for more than a lost crayon, and the child who is leaning against you for close inspection of your unusual earrings or holding on to your legs for dear life may not hear the directions for the next task. Limit setting and discretion deters distraction.

On a more serious note, many children will come to your classroom with a history of sexual abuse. Abuse of this nature often provokes a variety of responses toward teachers, ranging from extreme fear of being touched to overt seductiveness. It is frequently difficult, at first, to distinguish between a youngster's normal affection and sexual curiosity and sexual preoccupation and provocativeness. Over time, most of you will sense when a child is engaging you beyond the limits of normal affection. However, this is a complex problem to which I will only pre-alert you and strongly recommend that you bring it to the team's attention so that, together, you can formulate and implement a constructive treatment plan.

Recognizing Success

"I hope you won't take this personally, but. . . ." Think of these words whenever you are under a barrage of verbal abuse about your IQ, your mother, your looks, your family, or your intentions toward the youngster delivering the onslaught. The temptation is to respond in kind or retaliate with some immediate action to soothe your wounded ego. You try so hard, and this is what you get! When working with disturbed children, you have to learn, early, not to take their angry outbursts personally. This is not to say you condone their outbursts, but, in themselves, they are not a measure of your success or failure as a teacher. As has been said before, you are the nearest and, probably, the safest target at which to vent their feelings. So do not take their words personally.

You will learn to recognize the success of your team's work in the little changes that are made over time. Several examples follow:

> After 3 months, Vickie arrived one morning without her doll. Vickie no longer needs her transition object from home. She is now able to use the safe environment of your classroom for further development. Keith, who has torn up his math papers for months when you've tried to explain something to him, surprises you one day when he asks for help with division. One day you realize that Rob's time-outs have decreased from one every hour to about two a day.

Such shifts are indicators of success. Not to be attempted too soon, but you will really want to celebrate when you can leave the group unattended in the classroom long enough to go to the toilet, and upon your return, find everything in one piece. Success is a slowly emerging realization that a child is beginning to stand on his or her own ego instead of yours.

The Others versus You

Even the best of teacher-training programs will not prepare you for your initiation into a multidisciplinary treatment center with "the others." They include the clinical, teaching, and research staff (e.g., psychiatrists, psychologists, and social workers), with a variety of degrees (e.g., MDs, PhDs, EdDs, and MSWs); trainees such as child fellows, residents, interns, postdocs, teachers, and social workers; and a variety of consultants. They want to communicate so there are a lot of meetings and most of them speak in strange tongues. At least this will be your first impression, unless you were raised in the psychiatric model. You may find yourself carrying a psychiatric dictionary around with you to help translate the conferences concerning children who are scheduled to enter your group soon. These encounters with the others are terribly intimidating at first, and you risk beginning to think of yourself as an "eighthly"—the person lowest in the multidisciplinary hierarchy. There will be times when you feel you are the overseer of a holding pen (for cattle) from which the others take, use, and return. You seat yourself in the back row at these conferences and meetings and accept that you will be the last person to present your data at staffings and team meetings. You quickly adjust to the others when they ask you to change your class schedule to accommodate someone's therapy time or a parent conference.

It may be normal to feel like a stranger in alien territory at first; after all, this is a medical center, not a public school. How long you choose to remain an eighthly is up to you. Without you, there would be no day treatment program for emotionally disturbed children. Your expertise is as vital to the functioning of the center as anyone else's. Rediscover your sense of humor and polish up your self-esteem. If you remain an eighthly, it is because that is where you want to be.

THE TALE'S END

This cautionary tale has led you through an array of unpredicted experiences that you may encounter as you develop a working alliance with the children, their parents, and the staff of a psychoeducational treatment center. By prealerting you to expect the unexpected, some potentially traumatic situations may be defused, and you will be able to approach them from a clearer perspective. This, in turn, is likely to help you respond from a position of rigid flexibility, thereby ensuring a stable, predictable classroom environment.

Working with emotionally disturbed children is always challenging, often gratifying, and it can be fun if you keep firmly in mind that "If you haven't got a sense of humor, you haven't got any sense at all. . ." (Metcalf, 1987).

REFERENCES

Blom, G. E., & Parsons, P. C. (1976). The education of the emotionally disturbed child of elementary school age. In R. L. Jenkins & E. Harms (Eds.), *Understanding disturbed children.* (pp. 240–268) Seattle: Bernie Straub.

Blom, G. E., Rudnick, M., & Weiman, E. (1966). A psychoeducational treatment program: Implications for the development of potentialities in children. In H. Otto (Ed.), *Explorations in human potentialities.* Springfield, IL: Charles C Thomas.

Cohen, S. (1966). Teaching emotionally disturbed children. *Children, 13,* 232–236.

Cousins, N. (1979). *Anatomy of an illness as perceived by the patient.* New York: Norton.

Haring, N. G., & Phillips, E. L. (1962). *Educating emotionally disturbed children.* New York: McGraw-Hill.

Keelan, J. (1987). *Liven up your life with humor.* Arvada, CO: Communication Unlimited.

Kounin, J. (1970). *Discipline and group management in classrooms.* New York: Holt, Rinehart & Winston.

Long, N. J., & Newman, R. G. (1971). Managing surface behavior of children in school. In N. J. Long, W. C. Morse, & R. G. Newman (Eds.), *Conflict in the classroom: The education of children with problems.* Belmont, CA: Wadsworth.

Metcalf, C. W. (1987, June). *The humor option.* Paper presented at a 1-day seminar at the University of Colorado Health Sciences Center, Denver, CO.

8

The Cook, the Kitchen, the Cafeteria, and Beyond

Food in the Day Treatment Program

SARA GOODMAN ZIMET and GERALDINE F. SCHULTZ

INTRODUCTION

Food means many things to people. For some, it may conjure up negative experiences: It may have been an area of neglect in infancy or childhood as a result of economic deprivation and/or psychological or physical abuse; it may have provided the battleground for struggles between parents and children; it may be associated with allergies and other health-related matters; or it may represent the responsibilities of caring for others rather than being cared for by others. For many of the children in a day treatment center, there is a high probability that any one or more of these negative associations with food will be a reality. For most people, however, food is associated with good feelings, good tastes, and wonderful smells. Metaphorically, food represents having one's basic needs met even if they have not been met regularly or satisfactorily in the past.

A basic tenet of psychoanalytic thinking is that eating and being fed are synonymous with feelings of security, love, trust, and a sense of well-being (Erikson, 1950). Social and behavioral theories also recognize the

SARA GOODMAN ZIMET and GERALDINE F. SCHULTZ • The Day Care Center, Department of Psychiatry, University of Colorado Health Sciences Center, Denver, Colorado 80262.

impact of the experience of being fed and the role of food as a rein-
forcer in learning situations. Food has been used both to punish children
for bad behavior and to reward them for good behavior (Haworth &
Keller, 1962).

Traditionally, food has provided the reason for bringing people
together to celebrate an important event within a family or community.
Many religious and cultural rituals use the preparation and eating of
special foods, as well as the denial of favorite ones, as a way of expressing
beliefs and demonstrating practices. The preparation, serving, and eating of food at our day treatment center also has its traditions. It plays a
crucial role in contributing to the therapeutic atmosphere for the children and their families, as well as for the staff. At the same time that
nutritional needs are met, visual and olfactory senses are being stimulated, and oral and gastronomic pleasures satisfied. On many occasions,
food is used as the vehicle to bring people together to share in a common
purpose as well as to celebrate special occasions. It also serves as a motivation for learning when it becomes a part of the curriculum. While
planning a menu, purchasing the food and then cooking it, reading,
writing, and arithmetic skills are being applied, and a functional chem-
istry of turning liquids into solids and solids into liquids is observed. We
start with the cook, the kitchen, and the cafeteria, and we expand to the
classroom, the therapy room, and the meeting room. The many different ways that food enters our program and intersects with the lives of the
families we treat are discussed in detail next.

Nutritional Considerations

We know that the nutritive values in food prepared for children will
affect their growth and development. One nutritionist who has written
several books on the subject is quoted as saying that it is not what is in a
child's diet that relates to behavior problems, but what is missing from
that diet—the basic and important nutrients (McGuire, 1987). Nutrition
has always been a top priority in institutional cooking for children, and it
is strictly monitored by state departments of education (formerly by the
U.S. Department of Agriculture) in all settings participating in the Child
Nutrition Program. Under this program, each meal or snack served to a
child or adult must meet minimum nutritional standards described in
detail in their guidelines.

Food Preferences and Attitudes

It seems reasonable to assume that family experience should be a
major factor in the acquisition of food preferences and attitudes to

foods. Research with normal young children, however, has not justified this conclusion (Rozin, Fallon, & Mandell, 1984). It may be that the extent to which variety is introduced into the menu at home will influence most children's willingness to taste something new outside of the home. Another factor that may be influencing this level of risk taking for children attending our treatment center is that in most areas of their lives, the familiar and known is preferred to the unknown. Rejection of new foods, or of familiar foods prepared in new ways, is likely to be met by numerous nonverbal, verbal, and vocal expressions of rejection and disgust. Although dislikes for certain foods are not peculiar only to emotionally disturbed children, a larger number of food aversions has been reported by these children as compared to children who have fewer emotional and behavioral problems (Smith, Powell, & Ross, 1955). One would expect, therefore, that as treatment progresses, the children in day treatment would begin to show less aversive responses to food. Also, during their stay at the center, they would begin to associate the satisfaction of their hunger with feelings of well-being and security. In the words of Alexander (1953, p. 228), "For the child, to be fed is equivalent to being loved." As yet, however, there is no research to substantiate the belief that we can have a significant impact on the long-term food attitudes and behaviors of these children.

We believe, nevertheless, that trying new foods is likely to be affected by the children's attitude toward the person who prepares and serves the food (Lehman, 1949). In our situation, this person is our cook and kitchen manager. She is a sensitive, warm, and nurturing person with whom the children feel comfortable and by whom they are comforted. Although her primary role is preparing and serving them food, she is part of the total therapeutic program, and the children are aware of this. For example, periodically there are children who are either unable to settle down to any kind of classroom routine or who refuse to cooperate. We have had great success with some of these students by rewarding their cooperative behavior, at their request, with 15 minutes in the kitchen, before or after lunch, working with the cook. During this time, a child is expected to help with specific tasks: before lunch, setting out the empty trays by the steam table and placing the individual milk cartons, flatware, rolls, and napkins on each tray; after lunch, cleaning off the tables and chairs, wheeling the tray cart into the kitchen and placing the trays and flatware on the counter for washing, and wiping off the tray cart where food has spilled. Even in this short period of time, a child can accomplish a great deal and can feel satisfaction in a job well done. Accidents have happened but none that were not reversible; the atmosphere is nonpunitive and positive.

In addition to being a reward for appropriate classroom behavior, the children also see the cook in many other capacities: she provides ice cubes for bruised arms and legs; she dispenses and charts medication (under medical supervision); she plans and attends the family pot-luck dinner-meetings; she exchanges recipes with their parents; and she participates in the summer camp program. The children know that her expectations of their behavior are consistent with those of the rest of the center staff. Consequently, the children learn to trust her. Most of them eat their lunch and come back for second and even third helpings. These food enthusiasts also serve as an inspiration to the more hesitant ones and are often able to entice them to taste-test a new food item. We consider this to be a major accomplishment.

MEALTIMES

In inpatient settings, mealtimes have long been appreciated as having therapeutic implications (Herrmann, 1982). The extent to which food preferences and attitudes can be broadened and maintained by the environment outside the home, such as by friends, peers, and school lunch programs, remains a matter for speculation at the present time. We choose to believe, however, that in a day treatment setting, we can affect children in this area of their lives by setting the stage for making the eating experience at our center a pleasurable, instructional, and therapeutic one. We do this by (a) creating a calm, predictable, and attractive atmosphere in which to eat; (b) planning menus that combine sound nutrition and delicious food that children are likely to want to eat; (c) preparing and presenting food attractively; (d) having a sensitive, warm, and nurturing person as the cook and kitchen manager; and (e) providing mature and caring adults as table supervisors.

The Morning Snack

We have found that many of the children were having difficulty concentrating on the activities planned for them in the morning hours before lunch. We deduced that, in addition to the problem behaviors that brought these children to us, they were hungry. Sometimes the children do not eat breakfast at home, either because it is not prepared for them or they choose not to eat it. Even for those who do eat something, a fair amount of time elapses between the time they have had breakfast and their arrival at the center. This delay results in renewed appetites. These appetites may be stimulated even further by the 20 to

30 minutes of outdoor activities occurring between the time of arrival at the center and the time they start their morning activities.

In anticipation of the morning snack, the children eagerly enter the cafeteria and sit at designated tables with their teachers. The atmosphere is relaxed but orderly. The children are expected to socialize quietly and informally with one another while the snack is brought to their tables by one of their teachers. Along with fruit juice, buttered toast with jelly, cinnamon, or raisins is served most frequently. Occasionally, waffles, French toast, and zucchini or banana bread may be substituted. Some children have several helpings, whereas others eat more lightly. Within 15 minutes, they disperse to their group rooms, ready to concentrate on the primarily academic activities that follow. Even latecomers may stop by the kitchen for the snack that has been set aside for them without any serious disruption of their daily schedules.

Lunch at the Center

Lunch is included as part of the total therapeutic program and is considered to be a very important 30-minute block of time in the daily schedule. The activities centered around lunchtime present us with significant opportunities to develop trust and understanding, to teach the basic social skills needed when eating with others, and to intervene therapeutically. The children are brought to the lunchroom by their teachers, and they are expected to line up for their food trays in an orderly fashion. When their turn comes, the cook fills their tray with the minimum amount of food required by the Child Nutrition Program. Second and third helpings of food may be had up to 20 minutes into the half-hour. Before a child is served, she or he must be quiet, have eye contact with the cook, and be polite. The child then carries the lunch tray to one of the five tables to which he or she was assigned. The table supervisor is in the lunchroom to greet each child. Attentiveness to the children as they come from their classrooms often helps to set the tone for the entire lunch period. As the children finish eating, they bring their trays to a cart in the lunchroom, return to their tables, and remain there until dismissal time. They may take a detour to the resource table to find a quiet activity to engage in back at their lunchtable if they wish. The lunchroom supervisors are expected to be actively involved in these or other activities with the children.

Lunch Menus. Many of the children begin to ask, "What's for lunch?" when they arrive for their breakfast snack. We had capitalized on this curiosity about the lunch menu by having one child from each group report this information back to their class, either by word of mouth or by copying it from the cook's dictation or from a chart posted on the kitchen door. At other times, we will have one of the children who is especially interested or skilled make up a menu chart with food-item cards that they select from an alphabetized assortment.

The children do not have the option of bringing a sack lunch. We do have an occasional child who has certain dietary restrictions because of medical or religious reasons, and we work with the parents to provide the food that the child can eat. When our kitchen is unable to accommodate the family to their satisfaction, sometimes the solution is for the child to bring a sack lunch from home.

Favorite food items include hot dogs wrapped in fresh roll dough and baked, hamburgers, spaghetti, tacos, ovenfried chicken, and pizza. To the best of our knowledge, peanut butter and jelly pizza is original to our center. It came about from a conversation between the cook and some children who were wondering if it was possible to have such a "weird" topping on a pizza crust. The next time pizza was on the menu, the cook prepared both kinds: several of the traditional ones and one of the crust, only, which was spread with peanut butter and jelly. The result was "love at first bite." It has become a "tradition" at our center to make at least one pan of this open-faced sandwich whenever the old-fashioned pizza is served.

Along with the main course, we serve fresh fruit, a variety of raw vegetables and salads (canned vegetables are among the least favorite foods), and freshly baked bread. A bonus dessert of a freshly baked cookie may be earned by a child with appropriate lunchroom behavior.

Four Favorite Menus

Menu A
Beef tacos, corn, sopapillas with honey, applesauce, milk
Menu B
Barbecued chicken, tater-tots and salad, rolls, fresh fruit, milk
Menu C
Pizza, salad, fresh fruit, cookies, milk
Menu D
Cheeseburgers, parslied buttered potatoes, salad, fresh fruit, milk

Lunchtable Supervisors. Because lunchtime with disturbed and disturbing children may be fraught with tensions, steady and consistent staff supervision is of great importance (Evangelakis, 1974). We have provided this by placing a lunch supervisor at each of five tables, each table seating up to five children. It has been our experience that both children and supervisors benefit from permanent daily seating arrangements.

Each day of the week there is a different group of lunch supervisors. They are drawn from the center's clinical, research, and secretarial staff, from trainees in education, medicine, psychiatry, psychology, and social work, as well as from secretarial staff working in other parts of the medical center. Before meeting the children and being assigned a table, the supervisors undergo an orientation session where they are told about the needs of the children at our center, familiarized with the rules regarding the children's behavior, and given suggestions for how these rules are to be enforced. Tables are placed in close proximity to one another so that should a crisis arise, an experienced supervisor can be of assistance to the novice.

Lunchtime is a time for social interaction among children and adult lunch supervisors. Certain children will respond more readily than others to the table supervisor's efforts to engage them in positive verbal exchanges. However, as indicated earlier, mealtime is a period when tensions can be anticipated. For some children, the negative experiences that they have had regarding food may be played out repeatedly with the lunch supervisors and their peers. Abusing the food, swearing, making provocative comments or sounds, and starting fights are all to be expected at one time or another. Some prelunch experiences such as having had a difficult morning in class or missing a therapy session are likely to contribute to the child's disruptive or withdrawn behavior at the lunch table. Then there are the circumstances specifically related to the lunch activity that may cause problems for the children. For example, some children have difficulty in moving from one activity to another; this difficulty may be exacerbated when coming from a small group and room to the larger group and lunchroom. Furthermore, on some days, the table supervisor may be a child's psychotherapist, and the child may resent having to share this special person with the other children at his or her table.

Some of our children have had long-standing eating problems, either eating too much or not at all. Although all the children are expected to take a tray with food to their table and they are encouraged to taste their food, we do not get involved in food battles with them. In extreme cases, however, agreements are worked out among the child, the parents, and the child's team to change eating habits that may be detrimental to the child's health. The contract derived from this agreement is signed by all those mentioned, and the cook and lunch supervisors eating with the child are informed about the conditions to be met.

Lunchroom Rules. On the first day of the schoolyear and whenever necessary thereafter, a list of the following rules is presented to the children by the cook and the supervisors with the reasons for each rule:

1. Each child is expected to ask the supervisor for permission to leave the table.
2. Only one person at a table is to be away from the table at any one time.
3. Children are to talk to the people at their table only during lunch.
4. Games, books, and other materials taken from the resource table in the cafeteria after a child has finished his or her lunch are to be left at the lunchtable at dismissal time.
5. Children are to remain seated throughout the meal except to get second helpings, to return empty trays to the tray cart, to get something from the resource table, or to go to their next activity.

Infractions of rules are dealt with in a variety of ways depending on the seriousness of the infraction, the response of the child to being reminded of the rule, previous rule breaking by the child, and what is believed to be the most effective way of enforcing a rule with a particular child. An empathic comment about the child's concern may be enough to refocus the child's attention and behavior; directing the group in a general conversation about the issue at hand may help to calm the child; or redirecting the conversation to another topic that is less stimulating or anxiety producing may be a more effective intervention (Herrmann, 1982). Occasionally, a child's reaction may be of such a magnitude that he or she has to leave the lunchroom. The range of consequences might include a firm verbal reminder of the rules, a short time-out, a "standby" when the child is helped to calm down in the presence of another adult (see chapter where "Standby" is described in detail by Farley), finishing his or her lunch at a table alone in the hall or classroom, and/or missing dessert or "seconds." When a consequence is held over from one day to another, the child's readiness to return to a normal lunch period is determined jointly by the child's teacher, the table supervisor, and the child. As the supervisors get to know each child better, the behavior management approach that is most effective is discovered and used. If a lunch supervisor needs help in dealing with a child, assistance is at hand during the postlunch 20-minute "rehash" meeting that takes place everyday with the lunch supervisors and the cook.

Postlunch "Rehash" Meeting. One of the clinical staff who is supervising a table on that day is the designated discussion leader. At this meeting, notes are taken and entered in the child's clinical chart to provide continuity in carrying through on any changes in the lunch routine that may be recommended for a particular child. In this way, team members are kept apprised of factors that may be affecting a child's behavior. It is up to the cook to transmit any decisions made to the next day's table supervisors. This problem-oriented discussion provides a valuable learning opportunity for the trainees, many of whom only see the children in one specific setting or through the eyes of another staff member or parent.

FAMILY POT LUCK DINNERS

Twice each year, from 6:00 to 8:00 P.M., we have a pot luck dinner for the families and staff of our center. The turnout is always close to one hundred percent. The first one is held in December to celebrate the holidays. The second one is held in May to acquaint the parents with the summerschool camp program. All family members are invited—nuclear and extended as well as significant others. It is not unusual to find multiple parent combinations: step-mothers and step-fathers as well as biological parents and grandparents. Each year there may be one or two children who are unable to find the transportation to bring them to and from the center for this event. When this occurs, one of our staff will pick them up and take them back home.

Parents are asked to bring either a salad or dessert item to be shared with others; the center staff each brings a hot or cold vegetable side dish, relish plate, or appetizer to share; and the main course (cold cuts, hot dogs, rolls and bread), hot and cold beverages, dishes, flatware, cups, and napkins are supplied from the day care center budget. The setup and cleanup is also done by volunteers from the center staff. Approximately 90 people attend, and the cost to the center budget is approximately $50 for each dinner.

At the winter pot luck, we usually have entertainment from a community group interested in volunteering their time or willing to perform for a nominal fee. We have had magicians and musicians entertain us. At the spring dinner, we show the families a slide show about the camp where we take the children for 5 days at the start of our summerschool program (see chapter by Mulligan for a detailed description of this program). At both dinners we give away paperback books to each of the children as part of our association with the Reading Is Fundamental program (see chapter by Parsons and Imhoff for a description of this program). Each child is permitted to select three books for his or her own personal library.

FOOD IN PSYCHOTHERAPY AND COUNSELING

The offer of a cup of coffee and cookies to parents is a way of "breaking the ice" whether it be at their first intake interview or later on as a regular participant in the treatment program. This form of hospitality readily translates into the metaphor of a place where people care about people and one's needs are met.

Sometimes, when walking past the open kitchen door on the way up to a therapist's office, a parent may comment on the wonderful smells coming from the kitchen or on the positive attitude of the cook toward her work. These comments may lead directly into discussing issues concerned with being cared for by others and the responsibilities of caring for others, issues basic to having a child who is troubled and troubling and out of the mainstream.

Within a psychoanalytic framework, it is believed that food can be used to work through problems centering around orientation and reality testing, hostile—aggressive or masochistic tendencies, dependency conflicts, and the needs for love, security, trust, and acceptance (Haworth & Keller, 1962). Many children and adults find it easier to talk about a problem dealing with issues related to food when they are involved with food in some way. This involvement may be initiated by the therapists when they offer food to the child or adult in the therapy room. It also occurs on walks to the neighborhood convenience store when the therapist buys an edible treat for the child. Occasionally, however, a child and his or her therapist will decide to cook or bake something together during their therapy session. The preparation of the food is usually done in one of the therapy rooms down the hall from the kitchen; the baking is done in the kitchen oven that has been reserved in advance so that there is no conflict with the cook's food preparation activities.

CELEBRATIONS AND HOLIDAY PARTIES

Birthdays

Birthdays are always very special events for the children and are celebrated during the lunch period. For some children, they hold disturbing memories of the loss of parents through abandonment, divorce, or death, or of not ever having a fuss made over them on any occasion. Talk of parties at home and presents received for these children requires sensitive responses by staff.

Further complications arise when some parents ask to bring in very elaborate cakes for the school birthday party. This practice has upset those children whose parents do not do this. As a result, we have made it a policy for the center to provide the birthday cake to each of the children. The parents are told this when they enter their child in our program and are reminded of this policy if the question comes up again.

For most of our children, however, the birthday celebration offers them the opportunity to be special in a very positive way, and they thoroughly enjoy the attention focused on them. Each child's birthday is celebrated on the closest schoolday to their birthday. If it occurs during the long summer break, we schedule it on a day prior to the last day of school.

A special cake decoration with a single candle is placed on the piece of cake given to the birthday celebrant. We light the candle and everyone sings the happy birthday song after the child has made a wish and blown out the flame on the candle.

Thanksgiving Lunch

The week before Thanksgiving, we have a special luncheon for staff, trainees, therapists, and children. Turkey, potatoes, cranberries, hot rolls, and pumpkin pie are the main menu attractions. The children make festive placemats for all of the tables and special decorations that are hung around the room. Extra tables are set up in the gym/auditorium that adjoins the lunchroom. The children's food is served on their trays as usual; the adults help themselves buffet-style. It is the one day of the year that the children can sit at any table they choose.

Other Holidays

Halloween, Christmas, Chanukah (the Festival of the Lights), and Valentine's Day parties are held in the late afternoon of the designated day, just before the children leave for home. Refreshments are usually very simple: popcorn and fruit punch. These refreshments usually cap off a very stimulating day of parades, gift and card giving. The refreshments, at these times, provide the children with an opportunity to calm down while waiting for their rides home.

In addition to the parties, the children are likely to bake cakes or cookies with their teachers and decorate them with holiday motifs either to take home or to eat at school. Some cookies are hung as Christmas tree ornaments. They also are likely to prepare and cook potato pancakes as a classroom activity in celebration of Chanukah.

Halloween means carving pumpkins into jack-o-lanterns. The seeds are removed from the center, cleaned, and toasted in the oven for a special Halloween treat.

During Thanksgiving, two of the four groups assume the role of the Pilgrims, and each invites one of the other groups, who are the Indians, for an enactment of the first Thanksgiving feast. The Pilgrims prepare a variety of foods, such as cranberry relish, acorn and spaghetti squash, and corn bread—served with apple cider—and share them with the Indians, expressing their thanks for helping them to survive the first winter in the New World. The Indians, for their part, bring freshly made popcorn. In addition to providing the culminating experience to this social studies project, the children learn social skills involved in cooperating and in giving a party and practice the academic skills of arithmetic, writing, and reading. The teacher also reported that this project marked a turning point in the children's attitudes toward one another; it made them into a cohesive group.

The Center Cookbook. Several years ago we decided to compile a cookbook that would include recipes of favorite foods from the parents, the children, and the staff. Each child brings the cookbook home on the last day before the December holiday as a gift from our staff to the family. The book is attractively and humorously illustrated, typed by the office staff, and duplicated on our copy machine using pastel-colored paper. It has become a "tradition" and is added to each year in order to represent the tastes of our current population as well as those from the past.

Leaving Parties

On the child's last day at the center, we have a party during the lunch period. Ice cream and cake is served with the flavor selection being determined by the child. Chocolate cake with chocolate ice cream and strawberry cake with strawberry ice cream are most frequently requested. Flavors that are too off-beat for the group are discouraged and by this time, the child is usually willing to take this into account without making a fuss. Following dessert, the child who is leaving is presented with a special memory book containing photographs taken during his or her stay at the center and well-wishing notes from the staff and children. Parents often attend this party. The child is also presented with a special farewell gift from all the center staff.

THE CHILDREN AS COOKS

Cooking in the Classroom and the Kitchen

Cooking with their teachers, individual therapists, and with the cook, in the kitchen or in the classroom, has proven to be very successful for both the adults and the children at our center. It has been a non-bickering, cooperative joint venture. Creating something that smells good, looks good, and tastes good is, indeed, a rewarding experience for everyone. However, the younger children seem to be less concerned about the end product and are more focused on the process of preparing the food. The more activity involved in the preparation, the better. Rolling or pounding dough, tasting each of the ingredients, stirring, beating, and whipping, measuring, pouring, smelling, and feeling—all these activities are part of the cooking process that provides the children with the most gratifying part of cooking. Although these activities are important for the older children as well, they also care a great deal about the end product and want it to taste good and to look good as well.

When faced with the reality that a recipe has to be read to insure accuracy and success, reading takes on a new dimension. When children write out a shopping list based on a recipe, go to the store to purchase the food items needed, and follow the directions on the recipe, they are applying academic skills within a meaningful context. For some children, it may be the first time that they have made the connection between school learning and daily life functions.

Although large items are still baked in the kitchen, toaster ovens, crock pots, hot plates, and electric fry pans are used in the classrooms. Each classroom is equipped with its own cooking tools and containers.

Favorite Recipes

It seems appropriate to end this chapter with a selection of recipes that have proven to be useful with children between the ages of five and 12 years old and who are at varying developmental and ability levels. The recipes are not all foolproof, but this is seen as an advantage; mistakes that occur in a therapeutic setting can be very instructional, especially within the context of an activity where the process itself brings its own rewards.

Grape Jelly

Kids enjoy having something to take home.

2 cups of grape juice
$3\frac{1}{2}$ cups of sugar
$\frac{1}{2}$ bottle of fruit pectin

Mix sugar and juice together in a saucepan over high heat. Bring to a boil, stirring constantly. Stir in pectin at once and blend. Bring to a full boil and boil hard for 1 minute, stirring constantly. Remove from heat, skim off foam, and pour jelly into paper cups and cool.

Orange Delight

This is a big hit to serve midmorning.

$\frac{1}{4}$ cup orange juice concentrate

1 cup fresh squeezed orange juice

$\frac{1}{4}$ cup evaporated skim milk

$\frac{1}{2}$ cup skim milk

$\frac{1}{3}$ cup powdered sugar

2 teaspoons of vanilla

2 cups of crushed ice

Place all ingredients in a blender. Blend at high speed until frothy. Serve in chilled glasses. Makes two servings.

Quick Quiche Lorraine

The children were skeptical about "egg pie," but all took a bite and wanted more.

$\frac{1}{2}$ cup of bacon bits

$\frac{1}{2}$ cup of shredded Swiss cheese

$\frac{1}{4}$ cup of chopped onion

2 cups of milk

3 eggs

Place the first three ingredients on the bottom of a 9-inch-deep dish pie shell. Mix milk and eggs and pour on top of other ingredients. Bake at 375 degrees in an oven for 40 minutes.

Zucchini Bread

Easy to make and tastes great. The kids like shredding the zucchini.

3 eggs

1 cup of vegetable oil

2 cups of grated, raw, unpeeled zucchini

3 cups of flour

1 teaspoon of baking soda

1 tablespoon vanilla extract

1 cup of chopped nuts

Beat the eggs. Add the oil, sugar, and zucchini, and mix well. Stir in the flour and baking soda. Fold in the vanilla extract and nuts. Pour the batter into six small loaf pans. Bake at 350 degrees for 1 hour. Remove loaves from the pans and cool on a rack.

Fantastic Flapjacks

Lots of good measuring and good eating.
   2 cups of flour
   2 eggs
   $1\frac{1}{4}$ cups of milk
   3 teaspoons of baking powder
   1 tablespoon of honey
   $\frac{1}{4}$ cup of vegetable oil
Sift dry ingredients together. Beat eggs. Add honey and milk. Add vegetable oil. Mix only until the batter is smooth. Pour in small amounts onto griddle. Brown on both sides. Top with butter and honey, jelly, or syrup.

Indian Fry Bread

Kids enjoy using the rolling pin and making the holes.
   2 cups of flour
   4 teaspoons of baking powder
   $\frac{2}{3}$ cup of warm water
Combine flour and baking powder. Add water to make dough the consistency of bread. Pull off small pieces of dough and form into balls. Roll out each ball on a board lightly dusted with flour until the balls are flat and thin. Punch a hole in the center of each piece with your finger. Fry one at a time in 2 or 3 inches of hot vegetable oil. Drain on a piece of absorbent paper. Pour honey on top. Eat while they are hot.

The Gingerbread Man

There are lots of spices to smell.
   $\frac{1}{3}$ cup margarine
   1 cup brown sugar
   $1\frac{1}{2}$ cups molasses
   $\frac{2}{3}$ cup of cold water
   7 cups of flour
   2 teaspoons of baking soda
   1 teaspoon of allspice
   1 teaspoon of ginger
   1 teaspoon of cloves
   1 teaspoon of cinnamon
Mix first three ingredients. Stir in cold water. Sift together remaining ingredients and add to the above mixture. Roll the dough $\frac{3}{8}$-inch thick

and cut with a 5-inch gingerbread man cutter. Decorate with raisins and cinnamon candies. Bake at 350 degrees for 12 to 15 minutes in a lightly greased pan. Makes about 32 thin gingerbread men.

REFERENCES

Alexander, F. (1953). Emotional factors in gastrointestinal disturbances. In S. Portis (Ed.), *Diseases of the digestive system* (pp. 228–252). Philadelphia: Lea and Febiger.

Erikson, E. (1950). *Childhood and society.* New York: Norton.

Evangelakis, M. G. (1974). *A manual for residential and day treatment of children.* Springfield, IL: Charles C Thomas.

Haworth, M. R., & Keller, M. J. (1962). The use of food in the diagnosis and therapy of emotionally disturbed children. *Journal of the American Academy of Child Psychiatry, 1,* 548–561.

Herrmann, C. (1982). Mealtime. In J. L. Schulman & M. Irwin (Eds.), *Psychiatric hospitalization of children.* Springfield, IL: Charles C Thomas.

Lehman, E. (1949). Feeding problems of psychogenic origin: A survey of the literature. *The Psychoanalytic Study of the Child, 3/4,* 461–488.

McGuire, R. (1987, April 12). A little sweet-talk: Children's behavior tied to nutrition. *Rocky Mountain News Sunday Magazine.*

Rozin, P., Fallon, A., & Mandell, R. (1984). Family resemblance in attitudes to foods. *Developmental Psychology, 20,* 309–314.

Smith, W., Powell, E. K., & Ross, S. (1955). Manifest anxiety and food aversion. *Journal of Abnormal and Social Psychology, 50,* 101–104.

9

Beyond the City Limits

The Kids and Staff at Camp

PATRICIA MULLIGAN

INTRODUCTION

Our day treatment center at the University of Colorado Health Sciences Center has incorporated a 5-day camp experience into its yearly schedule for the past 15 years. The camp program provides the children and the center's staff members with a unique opportunity to get to know one another in a completely different kind of setting. In addition, well before the actual camp experience, it presents our clinical staff with an opportunity to work with the children and their parents on the important feelings associated with separation and independence. The camping experience itself, however, is viewed by our staff as a dramatic departure from the educational and therapeutic milieu of the group and individual work done during the rest of the year. We have learned over the years that in the recreational atmosphere of a magnificent mountain setting, it is possible to become motivated to learn a variety of social, athletic, and academic skills.

The success of our camp program can best be understood by listening to the children talk about it.

Here are some of their overheard comments: "I thought I would hate camp but I really had fun; I wish camp would last all year long; This is the first time I ever rowed a boat; Wait 'til my mom sees this fish I

PATRICIA MULLIGAN • The Day Care Center, Department of Psychiatry, University of Colorado Health Sciences Center, Denver, Colorado 80262.

caught!" Their eager anticipation of camp week and their enthusiastic participation in the camp program contribute to the accomplishment of the objectives established by the staff. Many of the children regard it as the highpoint of their school year and occasionally ask if they can attend camp even after completing their treatment at the Day Care Center.

This chapter will discuss the purpose and objectives of our camp program, describe various components of the program, and some of the practical considerations required for setting up an outdoor living experience for emotionally disturbed children. Although we recognize that there is an extensive literature on outdoor living and camping experiences for emotionally disturbed children, it is not the purpose of this chapter to review this literature.

PURPOSE AND OBJECTIVES

The main purpose of our camp program is to provide the children with an enjoyable, safe, and stimulating group experience away from the familiar surroundings of their home and our center, so that they can relate to each other and to the staff in a fresh context and learn the importance of sharing and cooperating. More specifically, the camp program is designed to help the children accomplish the following objectives:

1. To adapt to an unfamiliar environment.
2. To deepen their trust in their significant adult caretakers.
3. To develop mastery of new skills.
4. To increase self-esteem.
5. To increase peer social interaction and to develop new friendships.
6. To further the development of inner controls of their behavior and emotions in another setting.
7. To increase responsibility in self-care, problem solving, and group decision making in another setting.
8. To learn to be safe, healthy, and comfortable in outdoor surroundings.
9. To find satisfaction in learning to be better observers and participants in the natural environment.
10. To develop their appreciation of nature's beauty and the interdependence of all living things.
11. To grow in accepting the responsibility of caring for their environment.
12. To discover new ways to have fun!

PREPARING FOR CAMP

The Locale

Long before the sunny Monday morning in June when the trucks and station wagons pull out of the Day Care Center driveway on their journey to camp, preparations have been in the making for the big day. For 14 of the last 15 years, the DCC camp program has been held at Camp Santa Maria, a residential camp facility located in the Rocky Mountains, 60 miles west of Denver. Camp Santa Maria is operated by Catholic Community Services of the Archdiocese of Denver and is leased to us for 5 days each summer. The camp facilities are well-suited to the needs of this population of emotionally disturbed children. They include several dormitory cabins, a modern showerhouse with a separate area for toilets, a dining hall and kitchen, indoor and outdoor recreation areas, a fishing pond stocked with rainbow trout, a small lake with rowboats, hiking and nature trails, and a heated swimming pool. Riding stables and a refurbished ghost town are nearby. Leasing and financial arrangements are negotiated by our administrative officer during the winter months.

Staffing the Camp

Arranging staff participation at camp is the next project after finalizing the locale. In order to operate an effective camp program without overburdening any single segment of the staff, the expectation is that all of the staff members attend camp some of the time. Full-time staff are asked to participate for the 5 days, and part-time staff attend for 2½ days. This includes the director, assistant director, clinical social workers, research staff, teachers, classroom aides, cook, and some of the office personnel. In addition, special education practicum students and trainees in psychology, social work, and psychiatry, who are completing internships at the Day Care Center, often accompany the staff to camp as partial fulfillment of their training experience. The children's psychotherapists are also invited and encouraged to attend camp for as much time as they can manage. This visit, even if for only part of a day, has frequently proven to be an especially meaningful event for both parties.

This mixture of varied disciplines, talents, experiences, and perspectives provides a stimulating and enriching environment for both children and adults. However, an important component of camp preparation is the development of a unified approach toward fulfilling the purpose of the camp program. Individual philosophies must yield to the overall goal and objectives in order to provide the children with the consistency and stability they require.

Family and Staff Potluck Dinner

Another step in preparing for camp is the May potluck dinner, hosted by our center for the children and their families. All the families are encouraged to attend by their therapists, by the teachers, and, of course, by their children. Attendance is usually close to 100%. They are also encouraged to bring extended as well as immediate family members. Each family and staff member contributes a salad, side dish, or dessert, while our cook provides hot dogs and drinks (for a fuller description see the chapter by Zimet and Schultz).

The purpose of the dinner is twofold: (a) to bring the families and staff together in an informal nurturing atmosphere, and (b) to acquaint the children and their parents with the plans for the upcoming camp experience. At the same time the parents were invited to the dinner, they also were sent an informational letter regarding the camp purpose, dates, location, activities, and lists of clothing and equipment the children will need. This dinner-time gathering offers the opportunity for the camp director to answer the parents' questions and to comment on particular aspects of the letter that need to be emphasized, such as packing enough cold-weather clothes or making special provisions for the children's medical care. The culminating activity of the evening is the slide show of pictures from the previous year at camp, set to music. Because over one-half of our children are camp "veterans," having attended camp for at least one summer, there is much squealing and pointing as familiar faces are seen on the screen. A wealth of memories flood campers and staff members alike as they watch slides of all the fun, exciting, adventuresome, silly, and solemn camp activities. The parents, too, are generally struck by the beauty of the mountain setting and the wide range of activities in which their children participate. At least one or two parents comment each year on how much they would enjoy spending a week at camp as well. Although one picture may be worth a thousand words, our collection of slides says it all!

Although each class has talked about camp many times throughout the school year, the potluck dinner and slide show truly mark the beginning of our camp season.

The Preview Trip

The next preparation step is a 1-day preview trip to camp, which takes place sometime during the last 2 weeks of May. The cook prepares a picnic lunch, and the teachers drive university vehicles loaded with the excited and nervous soon-to-be campers. The purpose of the preview trip is to acquaint the children first-hand with the camp setting and to allay some of their fears. Because many of the children have never spent time in the mountains or away from home, they are full of questions and anxieties about wild animals, nighttime, the woods, the river, the food, toilet and shower facilities, and "who's going to watch me?" During the car ride, the teachers provide books and activities that emphasize getting along in the out-of-doors. Once at camp, the children's apprehensions manifest themselves in a variety of ways: withdrawal, braggadocio, silly laughter and behavior, and flaunting the rules in order to test limits. The children are given a brief tour of the camp and shown the in-bounds and out-of-bounds areas. After the picnic lunch and some free time on the camp's playground, it is time for the return trip to our center.

Learning Some Camping Skills

Another time-tested preparation step is to teach some outdoor living skills while the children are still at school. When a team of two children learns to pitch and strike a tent, for example, two goals are served: (a) the children gain a sense of mastery in this new arena, and (b) staff members know they will have one fewer task to do on the overnight campout. A mighty motivator for the campers learning to set up their own tent is the knowledge that at camp no other fun activities can take place until it is accomplished. Other examples of precamp skill learning are choosing appropriate clothing and footwear for a hike, gathering firewood, and rolling a sleeping bag. These assignments are met with much enthusiasm, and the children eagerly participate as the reality of camp draws closer.

Addressing Concerns about Bed-Wetting

Bed-wetting is a common area of concern for many of our children and their parents. The teaching and clinical staff discuss this problem with them before the children go to camp, assuring them that they are not alone in their concern but that we expect to help them with the problem while they are at camp. Most of the campers who are worried about bed-wetting are relieved to have the topic discussed in this matter-of-fact manner and are willing to work with us to determine what interventions would be most helpful. Some children have asked that they be awakened and taken to the toilet during the night; some stated that they would like plastic sleeping bag liners; others asked to be reminded not to drink liquids after dinner. The staff reinforces these problem-solving efforts. However, if all efforts fail to keep them dry through the night, we tell the children what they need to do when they wet the bed. Because there is a washing machine and dryer on the camp grounds for our use, they are expected to bring their own wet pajamas and sleeping bags to the laundry room where a staff member will take care of them. In addition to relieving the children's and parents' anxieties, we believe that by discussing the problem beforehand and by including the children in the solution, there has been a decrease in bed-wetting episodes at camp.

Medical Concerns

Our children come to camp with a variety of special physical conditions and medication regimens. For example, over the years, there have been campers with hemophilia, asthma, seizure disorders, allergies, and kidney dysfunction. Rarely has a child been prohibited from attending camp because of medical reasons. The staff, along with the child and parents, have exerted special efforts to ensure that medical needs are taken care of at camp, ranging from complete nightly peritoneal dialysis to nebulizer treatments for asthma. In addition, one of our staff members is assigned to dispense daily medications. This is no small task because between 30% and 40% of our children take some form of medication, either to control their medical condition or behavior, and, at the time they are to be given their dosage, they may be found anywhere from the swimming pool to the middle of the lake in a rowboat.

Aside from ongoing medical needs, the staff must be prepared for minor illnesses, sunburn, insect bites, and occasional injuries. In addition to a very complete first-aid kit, we have excellent medical coverage by our center's director who is a physician and who is at the camp for the 5 days.

Equipment and Supplies: Staff Responsibilities

Every staff member's assistance is needed to get things ready for camp. Materials need to be gathered, checked, repaired, purchased, and packed during the week before we leave for camp. Fishing equipment, basketballs, VCR and movies, insect repellent and craft supplies, tents, backpacks, and extra sleeping bags—these are just a few of the items that we will need at camp. One staff member makes up a folder for each child containing a variety of quiet activities to be used by early morning risers. Another assembles all the children's medications and dosage instructions. Another is in charge of gathering our nature supplies. With everyone's effort, we are prepared for most any activity in most any weather.

CAMP DEPARTURE DAY

Saying Goodbye

Finally the big day arrives. The scene at our center playground is one of controlled chaos. Staff, campers, and parents arrive with suitcases, backpacks, fishing rods, bedrolls, tents, and boxes of equipment varying from first-aid supplies to crafts materials. The staff's two main jobs are to pack the truck and to assist the families in saying goodbye. The range of emotions exhibited as parents and children prepare to spend 5 days apart is striking to watch. Some families cling to each other tearfully until the last possible moment; others manage only a quick hug and farewell; still other campers, looking forlorn, are not delivered by their parents at all but dropped off by public or private transportation services. We have found that this is a crucial time to be available for support to both the parents and the children, answering questions and reassuring nervous family members. Then, with a wave and a honk, the caravan is off.

The First Orientation Meeting

The children's orientation to the camp program occurs after the campers and staff members have settled into their assigned cabins and have had their first noon meal.

The Symbol of Togetherness. At this time, the camp director passes out caps or T-shirts emblazoned with the DCC camp logo to each camper and adult. These are not used as a uniform but rather as a symbol of the camp experience, a reminder that "We're all in this together."

The Symbols of Success. Also, at this time the children are shown a three-part banner, each section a different color, inscribed with the words *Discoverer, Ready Helper,* and *Friend Maker.* A staff member explains that as the group learns to live together in a cooperative way at camp, each child will have opportunities to excel in each of these areas. These three goals represent, in a simplified way, the underlying structure of the camp week and help the children to focus their energy through all the activities of each day. They are encouraged to report their successes (e.g., discoveries, new friends, times when they willingly helped out) to their group leaders and to each other. The banner, with its message, is one element of the positive behavior management system the staff employs at camp.

To help campers focus their energy in a positive direction, we have devised a system of awards that reinforces appropriate behavior and encourages cooperation among the campers. The children each receive a leather thong necklace on the first day of camp, and each day a camper may earn a large colored wooden bead to add to his or her necklace. The bead's color determines if it is an award for being a Discoverer, Ready Helper, or Friend Maker. In addition, campers may earn a large feather (a mock eagle feather) if they have been identified as being an all-around good camper for that day. The awards are presented at the campfire each night by one of our staff members who has conferred earlier with all the small-group leaders. As camp week progresses and the necklaces become more adorned with beads and feathers, the children become more motivated to participate enthusiastically and appropriately in the camp activities.

The Activity Group Assignments. The children and staff also are assigned to their activity groups at this time. The small groups (five to six children with two to three adults) are usually identical to the school classroom groups, with the same teacher and teacher aide plus additional staff. This is the basic operating unit that each camper functions within during camp week. The children and adults in each group work together to plan and implement their choices of activities for each day. Favorite activities chosen by each small group at least once during the week include fishing, hiking, boating, swimming, and hiking and nature exploring. In addition, indoor activities such as crafts, music, and games offer a change of pace and are a boon on rainy days.

The small-group format has also proven to be the most effective method of insuring continuous supervision of the children. Each small group has enough staff members assigned to it so that the campers are accompanied in all camp areas.

BEHAVIOR MANAGEMENT

We have found that the beautiful natural surroundings of the camp have great appeal for most of the children. They keep busy and interested with little time to spend on inappropriate behavior. In addition, of course, we have taken several steps toward structuring what we call a preventive rather than a reactive approach to behavior management. In this way, we feel that we are able to head off problems before they occur.

Supervision

The simplest yet most effective step that covers all activities at camp is that children are always to be with and supervised by an adult. Children are not allowed to be unaccompanied by an adult at a camp area (such as the boat house, fishing pond, swimming pool, cabin, or shower house), nor are they to begin an activity (such as boating, fishing, hiking, or showering) unless there is an adult present. Most of the problems in the past have occurred when children have wanted to move from one activity to another or have needed to return to the cabin area to change clothes or to use the toilet. This has resulted frequently in mischief and mayhem.

Clear and Consistent Expectations and Interventions

Our small-group leaders have found that the children's compliance increases when rules and expectations are clear and consistent and when reinforcement (positive and negative consequences) is immediate. When a child refuses to comply, the following hierarchy of interventions is implemented by the adult who is supervising:

1. Attempts to redirect the child's activity with the idea that a change of focus will engage the camper back on a positive course.
2. Attempts to defuse the problem by having the child remove him- or herself from the situation.
3. Prescribes a time-out.
4. Restrains the child who is not responding to verbal direction and who is in danger of hurting self or others.

HIGHLIGHTS OF THE WEEK

Nature Activities

One highlight of the week at camp is the children's interest and eager involvement in nature discoveries. The campers are encouraged to become close observers of their environment and to develop an appreciation of outdoor beauty and the interdependence of people and nature. This awareness does not occur by osmosis or by merely putting children into the outdoor environment. Our staff takes an active role in teaching children to observe and wonder about their surroundings and provides opportunities for exploring and questioning. Some examples of large group structured nature activities are (a) a scavenger hunt, where each team is challenged to find as many listed items as possible; (b) an ABC nature hike, finding an item for each letter of the alphabet; and/or (c) a riddle hike, locating natural objects when only a clue is given. In addition, the small-group leaders informally point out and discuss with the children natural phenomena as they appear during the course of the week's activities. Resources such as books on birds, mammals, trees, and insects are kept in the main recreation hall for handy reference after a hike.

The children are encouraged to bring back samples of their discoveries to a designated area in the indoor recreation building. With the help of the adults, they label them and display them for the week. They are cautioned against disturbing an animal's habitat or picking wildflowers. By the end of camp, the display table is filled with such fascinating Rocky Mountain wonders as pinecones; seeds; animal bones, teeth, hair, and antlers; rocks; insects; and bird feathers, bones, and nests that have fallen out of trees. Crafts projects also are designed to capitalize on outdoor interests and the children's curiosity. Paperweights are made from colorful pebbles, stones, and from casts of animal footprints; tongue depressors and feathers found on hikes become bald eagles or fantasy birds; butterflies are made from tissue paper and a clothespin.

All Campers and Staff Activities

Complementing the daily projects of the small groups are several activities that involve all the campers and staff members. Everyone joins in the evening hikes, campfires, outdoor games, and horseback riding.

The Overnight Campout. The all-camp event that is anticipated most anxiously (both eagerly and "worriedly") is the overnight campout, truly a highlight! This is planned for the third night of camp, after the children have become comfortable with the camp structure and with their responsibilities within their small groups. As plans for the campout are discussed, the camp director again emphasizes the cooperative attitude that is vital to the success of such a large-scale venture. A staff member demonstrates how to pack appropriate clothing and equipment for spending a night out-of-doors. Staff and children return to their cabins and assist each other in packing for the overnight.

Because carrying all the gear in backpacks has proven to be a major effort without substantial rewards, the children and staff are offered the choice of either backpacking their personal gear or having it delivered by truck to the campsite. The staff and some children help in loading tents, food, and all the necessary supplies on the truck.

During the 2-mile hike to the campsite, many questions arise again about bears, ghosts, tornados, and other worrisome things. Even the oldest and boldest campers listen carefully as staff members address these concerns. Upon arrival at the campsite, the first order of business for each camper is to choose a tentmate and pitch their tent together. We have found that when more than two children are assigned to a tent, friction is the likely outcome. As our "tent city" is erected in the mountain meadow, time is provided for the children to explore this new environment. They may play appropriately in their tents, or they may investigate the nearby stream and woods with staff members.

The small-group leaders call the campers together again for wood gathering and for an optional hike to an abandoned cave before dinner. Meanwhile, two staff members prepare the campfire and heat the hobo dinners that have been assembled in the morning in the camp kitchen. Each hobo dinner includes meat and a vegetable and is wrapped in aluminum foil and cooked over the campfire. The dinner is served with chips, a beverage, and dessert. After dinner and the ritual campfire activities, it is bedtime. Bedtime for these children means that each is able to place a great deal of trust in his or her environment, in him- or herself, and in our staff. This trust is aided somewhat by the presence of each camper's trusty flashlight. However, by this time in the week, the batteries are likely to have been severely taxed, and the lights produced barely pierce the deep mountain darkness. Suddenly it seems as though there are strange sounds previously unnoticed during daylight hours. A tent seems a flimsy home indeed against such fears as falling meteorites and wild animals. A camper's best friend suddenly is his or her tentmate, who, one hopes, does not fall asleep first. Some staff members are called into more direct service to comfort a child. The voices of the adults laughing and talking late around the campfire also provide reassurance. Mastering this challenge is indeed a very big step toward building the confidence of all of our campers. And they all make it!

Dawn's early light illuminates a grimy and bedraggled group of children who have boundless energy and amazing stories of nighttime bravery to share. Our staff has not yet discovered a foolproof way to keep the 6 o'clock risers from awakening those who would like a bit more rest, so everyone is off to an early start. Hot chocolate, oatmeal, and English muffin/ham/melted cheese sandwiches never tasted so good as on a chilly morning in the mountains, and we bless the hardy soul who built the fire. The bed-wetters get help in drying out themselves and their sleeping bags; then we turn to the morning's main tasks: (a) packing up tents, cooking equipment, and personal gear; and (b) cleaning up the campsite. We notice each year that some children are able to take care of their things plus cheerfully assist with other jobs, whereas some campers need help just to gather their own belongings. When the truck, backpacks, and canteens are loaded up, the children and staff begin the speedy hike down the mountain.

After the Overnight

The remaining 2 days and 1 night at camp are deliberately kept low-key. Available activities include swimming (encouraged right after returning from the campout for the sake of cleanliness), quiet cabin activities, and a VCR movie in the evening after our campfire. By the final morning, the children's attention focuses on thoughts of home, and packing, cleaning, and truck loading are the main tasks. The Day Care Center camp comes to a close after the final lunch and presentation of individual awards.

RITUALS AND CEREMONIES

The Campfire

The nightly campfire is just one of several ceremonial events that provides the children with opportunities for reflection. The ceremonial traditions also provides a rhythm to the week's activities and a predictability that is comforting to the children. The camp director gathers the campers and staff at the fire ring and includes these features each night in this same order: a snack, singing, awards, joining hands to sing *Taps*, and dismissal to the cabins for the night. If the director inadvertently leaves out any part of the campfire ceremony, the children are sure to call it to his or her attention, emphasizing again, for the staff members, the importance of the ritual.

The Wish Boat Float

On the final night of camp, the children and staff participate in the Wish Boat Float. This tradition is designed to help the campers reflect on their week at camp and the growth they each have made. During the day, each child makes a "boat" from a cut-down half-pint milk carton with a small vigil candle attached by clay to the inside bottom. The staff member in charge helps the children review their experiences at camp and encourages them to recall the good decisions they have made, the problems they have helped to solve appropriately, the new friends they have made, the fears they have overcome, or the wishes they might want to express. These are written on small cards, folded, labeled with each child's name, and stapled to the side of the milk carton boat. At dusk that evening, the campers proceed to the fishing pond, light their candles, and set their boats afloat as the camp director leads the group in song. Within minutes, the boats appear to be only flickering lights bobbing gently on the waves, and even the most cynical camper is momentarily silenced.

REST AND RELAXATION

We have found that scheduling time for rest and relaxation reduces the stress of camp week for both our children and staff members. Although the greater part of each day is spent in structured activities, the small groups also schedule in some free time for playing in the playground area or just hanging out in their cabins. Before camp week begins, one staff member makes up a folder for each child containing a variety of quiet activities. This "bunktime folder" holds small sets of crayons and markers, coloring pages, dot-to-dots, mazes, word puzzles, and drawing and writing paper. The campers may choose to use these during free time, during the afterlunch rest hour, at bedtime, or early in the morning before their cabinmates awaken.

In addition, we participate in the Washington, DC-based Reading Is Fundamental (RIF) program, which helps to provide discounted paperback books for our children to keep. To help wind down after the overnight campout, one of our staff members displays an assortment of books for the children to browse and choose one to take back to their cabins for the rest hour and then take home with them at the end of camp.

One more responsibility of the camp director is the prevention and care of staff exhaustion. Staff members are encouraged to monitor their own energy levels and take some time away from the children. Break times are arranged among the adults in each small group to ensure continued supervision of the children.

Our staff members who chose not to participate in the overnight campout are expected to assume responsibility for helping the children to unpack, take showers, and wind down upon their return to their cabins. The campout staff, then, has some well-earned time to freshen up and relax.

Another source of relaxation for our staff is the nightly "staff meetings" held after the children are in bed. A rotating skeleton crew is left to supervise the cabins while the rest of us relax in front of the fireplace in the recreation hall with our peers, pretzels, and a variety of other refreshments.

As demanding as these 5 days are on everyone's stamina and patience, there are several enticing incentives for those of us who persevere. First and foremost is the positive effect it appears to have on the children. Second, each of us is given compensation in the form of 2 vacation days for each day we spend at camp, in effect, providing us with rest and relaxation (R and R) at a place of our own choosing.

CONCLUSION

For 15 years, the camp experience has held a unique place in the Day Care Center's program. The children themselves have told us and shown us in so many ways how important it is to them. They have demonstrated progress in making friends, in working within a group, in conquering fears, in learning about the outdoors, in becoming more independent, and in mastering new skills. Whenever our staff wonders about the value of camp because of its cost or because of the drain on our energy, we remind ourselves of its positive impact on the children we serve.

Special Projects in the Treatment Program
Their Birth, Development, and Occasional Demise

PHYLLIS C. PARSONS and RALPH IMHOFF

INTRODUCTION

This chapter is aimed at describing, in detail, some of the special projects that have been introduced to the Day Care Center treatment program over the 26 years of its existence. We refer to them as *special* because they have been additions to our regular program and were adopted to meet specific therapeutic needs of the children and, at the same time, to introduce novelty and excitement into the program for the benefit of the children and the adults. None of the projects was suggested directly by the children themselves. They emerged, indirectly, however, from observations of the children by staff members, who then took the initiative to design a project that would address a persistent interest, meet a need, or solve an emerging problem. Occasionally, however, it would work the other way around: A staff member would hear about the opportunity of adopting an interesting project and check to see if it would be of value to our special group of children. Many of them were aimed primarily at improving a variety of academic skills (e.g., Reading Is Fundamental, Movement Activity Reading Program, Listening Project, Stamp-ing Around the Country, Practicing the Three Rs, and Automechanics);

PHYLLIS C. PARSONS and RALPH IMHOFF • The Day Care Center, Department of Psychiatry, University of Colorado Health Sciences Center, Denver, Colorado 80262.

whereas others focused on improving social skills, facilitating the transition from our center to a community school, imparting knowledge, increasing understanding about self and others, and enjoying music (e.g., Making Friends, Field Day/Festival Day, The Structure and Function of the Human Body, People-to-People Study and Travel, and Folk Singing). In truth, however, each served a multitude of purposes and contributed to various areas of the children's development, social, emotional, physical, and academic.

Some of these projects have had a short life span for any one of the following reasons: (a) our basic program changed in some significant way so as to render a project obsolete; (b) the need for which a project was originally adopted could be met more effectively in some other way, possibly through the adoption of another project; (c) the project's start-up funds were obtained from an agency outside of our treatment center, and our operating budget was not sufficient to continue it without these funds; (d) the staff members who were expected to carry out the project were not the ones who had initiated it; (e) the staff members who had assumed responsibility for its continuation had left, and there was no one to take their place; (f) the responsible staff member became bored with the project; (g) the project did not work; (h) the project interfered with other parts of the program; and/or (i) a project needed a broader base of staff support and did not get it.

On the other hand, some special projects have withstood the test of time and have become an integral part of our treatment program. Their longevity may be attributed to the ease with which they could be adapted to changes in our overall program goals or to the economic viscissitudes that befell us over the years.

In the following pages, some examples of both the short- and long-lived projects are described. Perhaps these descriptions will serve as a stimulus to those of you who are looking for ways to meet basic program needs in a new way in order to introduce novelty into your program; or perhaps they will furnish you with the foresight to keep you from adopting a project where the payoff is likely to be minimal.

Field Day/Festival Day

The year was 1973. The children were bedecked with ribbons; family and staff members autographed pupil-made yearbooks and lined up for the grand finale—a hot dog roast. Another Festival Day was about to become history. When had it all begun?

In the Beginning. The first such event was held at the end of the Day Care Center's second year of operation, in June 1964. At that time, it was

called Field Day rather than Festival Day. Our policy had been to graduate all the children at the end of 2 years, and Field Day was the culminating event—a sort of graduation party. Because Field Day was a tradition
in the community schools from which the children came and to which
they would return, we believed that this activity created a link between
our center and these schools that would make the move for the children
and their families easier. Thus, initially, Field Day events were patterned
after those in the regular schools. They included competitive activities
such as ball throws, broad jumps, high jumps, and various types of
individual and cooperative team sports. The team sports were judged on
the basis of first and second place, with each team member receiving a
first- or second-place ribbon. In the individual competitions, the few
children who were athletically skilled won most of the ribbons in these
events. Therefore, we also included activities that focused on such accomplishments as the amount of effort expended, the amount of improvement that took place in a skill over the 2-year period, and the
willingness to participate. There also were a few activities that called for
the "luck of the draw" rather than skill. In effect, we had our own Special
Olympics in which everyone was assured of receiving at least one ribbon.

Following on the heels of the competitive events was the signing of
autographs in each child's hand-made autograph book. This, too, was a
tradition of the regular schools and would serve our children as a link to
all the people, children, and adults who had played a significant role in
their lives over the past two years. This, also, was seen as a transitional
object, one that would counterbalance, to some extent, any feelings of
loss they might experience.

While autographs were being signed, the smell of hot dogs cooking
on the outdoor grill began drawing the participants and observers toward
the food tables. Families and staff members sharing this informal but
celebratory "breaking of bread" marked both an end and a beginning.

As Things Began to Change. As our entry and length-of-treatment
policy became more flexible, the characteristics of graduation day
changed as well. Children were accepted at various times during the year,
and the duration of their treatment varied between 1 and 3 years. Some
children left (were graduated), whereas others stayed on at the center. In
addition, many of the staff members were uncomfortable about the
strong emphasis on competitive athletic activities, with either sparse or no
attention given to the children's other accomplishments. It was at this time
that the culminating event underwent a major redefinition. As a result,
Field Day was transformed into Festival Day, which became a yearly event.
It continued to include the competitive events described earlier as well as
displays throughout the building of the children's schoolwork, pho-

tographs taken at special events, and art and crafts activities. This involved storing material for these displays throughout the year. For example, it was not uncommon to say of a youngster's Halloween project, "Let's put this in the storeroom to use for Festival Day in June."

The other major transformation occurred with the autograph book; it became a yearbook, highlighting each child's year at the center. It included favorite drawings, interviews, hobby pages, and a host of reports on favorite foods, TV programs, and liked and disliked events in which each had participated. Teachers began to assume too much responsibility for children's projects, and the yearbook became such a production that it was doubtful a youngster could recognize his or her own contributions.

The modifications that took place changed the very nature of the culminating event from a special day every second year, to an attempt to highlight a whole year. What had taken 1 month's preparation once every 2 years was now taking 9 months every year. What had been planned as a way of creating a smooth transition, a nostalgic review of the past, and a therapeutic focus on a new beginning, became an obsession with a single future event. It seemed that, like a balloon, this event grew so big that it finally burst, and with its "pop," children and staff were relieved of unintentionally imposed pressures.

The New Culminating Event. The need for which Field Day/Festival Day was meant to serve took on a different character, although a few remnants still exist. There are no competitive athletic events. The recognition ceremony of the child's departure occurs at lunch; the child's parents are invited to come. Following lunch, the child receives a memory book and a gift from all the staff. The memory book includes well wishes from staff members and children in the program. In addition, it holds a small collection of photographs taken of the child alone or with other children and staff during the child's tenure at the center. (See the description in the Zimet and Schultz chapter.)

The responsibility of creating a smooth transition for the children and their families rests more heavily on other aspects of the program (see "Ending Day Treatment" in this chapter). In addition, informally breaking bread with the children and their families occurs at our twice-yearly pot luck dinners (this is described in the Zimet and Schultz chapter).

Thus the demise of Field Day/Festival Day was greeted with cheers from the staff. Shifting from a highly charged, pressured event to low-keyed, easily accomplished ones truly marks a new beginning for the staff, children, and parents without sacrificing other important program components.

Ending Day Treatment: Let's Talk about It

Introduction. The capacity to adapt is the key to survival in the regular school classroom. Emotionally disturbed children have a limited response repertoire and tend to use the same maladaptive behaviors to meet most situations. A primary treatment focus at the Day Care Center, therefore, is on helping children to replace maladaptive with adaptive responses to a variety of real-life situations. Although there is no difficulty in finding daily challenges for children and staff to work on throughout their attendance at the center, one very critical experience that puts all that effort to a final test occurs during the final few months of treatment. Here is a typical scenario:

> The treatment team has decided that Brad is ready to return to a regular school. Brad and his family have been part of that decision. But, as the end approaches, the atmosphere around this child is charged. For example, the teachers expected more of Brad than of the other children in his class—expecting him to behave as though he were already in the regular school by raising his hand before speaking, taking pride in his paperwork, and not provoking fights with the other children during free play. On the other hand, while Brad was initially pleased about leaving, he is now experiencing a combination of other feelings, such as sadness, anxiety, and anger. In fact, many of the behaviors for which he had been referred to day treatment have resurfaced. Behavior crises are the norm for Brad, and it was discouraging for his teachers, other concerned staff, and his parents to relive the old problems. However, staff members also recognize that this typical reaction to leaving the security of the Day Care Center provides a wealth of material that can be used to strengthen Brad's capacity to adapt.

The Old Way of Leaving. In the course of treatment planning for all children, ending treatment at the Day Care Center was dealt with by each child in individual therapy, and by the treatment team making the necessary contacts with the child's home school. This process usually covered several months. When an appropriate placement was found in the child's home school district, the child's teacher accompanied the child on a visit to the receiving school and classroom, and, whenever possible, the child gradually increased the amount of time spent in the new setting while decreasing the time spent in our center. More often than not, the child lived in a community far from our center and transportation problems made a gradual transition difficult or impossible. The process had to be speeded up, therefore, and went from one or more visits to the school, to full time in the new program. Reentry problems had to be solved in outpatient therapy if the child continued treatment or by telephone.

Some of us thought that we might be able to improve on this transition model, so we came up with the one described next.

The New Way of Leaving. Four to 5 months prior to terminating day treatment, the six or seven children scheduled to leave were grouped together, regardless of age, for academic class time during the morning. They were called the Transition Group and were in a separate classroom. Children in this Transition Group knew they were leaving the treatment center and that they would be returning to a situation in which most had experienced failure and defeat. Although most of the children were aware that their behaviors and coping skills had improved, they needed to find out how capable they actually were in transferring what they had learned to a previously hostile environment. This new model of leaving, in effect, was aimed at providing the children with an enriched and supportive pathway to the real world and an opportunity to share common problems with peers in a similar situation. In order to accomplish this, we used the components described next.

Placing the Children in a Transition School. We decided that the move to the children's home schools would be preceded by placement in a school within walking distance of the treatment center. In this way, the children could keep a foot in both doors, the one at the center and the other at the transition school, starting with as little as 1 hour a day in the receiving classroom and increasing the amount of time until they were full time.

Maintaining Communication with the Transition Schoolteacher. Continuous communication was maintained, either through classroom observation and consultation or by telephone, with the neighborhood school by the transition group teacher and staff social worker assigned to work with these children. We chose to observe for several reasons: (a) to find out how the children performed in a large group; (b) to assure the teacher, by our presence that we were not simply dumping a troublesome youngster in their classroom but were there for consultation if needed; and (c) to be better equipped to inform parents of their children's adjustment. We were told that we were welcome to observe at any time, but we always arranged our visits beforehand. Not infrequently, teachers would ask us to observe another child with whom they were having trouble, and, frequently, we would consult with them about that child rather than the one from our center. Many of the problems we were asked about were fairly routine ones, such as excessive talking, failure to complete assignments, or refusing to participate. With rare exceptions, we found that the teachers wanted either advice on how to manage a situation or reassurance about their methods of dealing with these annoyances. Their main concern was that their methods might be harmful because the children were still in a treatment setting. Several examples come to mind. Once we were called about a fourth-grade girl who constantly masturbated in class. The teacher did not know how direct she should be in discouraging this behavior. At our center we had told the child, matter-of-factly, to keep her hands on her desk. The teacher felt comfortable in adopting this approach. Another time, one of our children was caught red-handed as she was going through her classmates' coat pockets and keeping various objects for herself. According to school rules, this behavior resulted, automatically, in a 2-day suspension. Instead of automatically invoking the rule, however, we were called to meet with the teacher and principal to determine how they should deal with the situation. The child was still expected to conform to the school's rules, but a clear statement of the policy was made to the child, and she was assisted in returning the stolen items to her classmates. In addition, we spent time discussing the problem in the transition group's rap sessions at the center (see "Rap Sessions").

Parallel Classroom Structures. We structured our new classroom at the center more like those found in the regular schools. For example, we expected everyone to wait their turn before speaking, to do more written work using specific formats, and to do homework assignments.

Rap Sessions. Three times a week, we held rap sessions, scheduled for 45-minute periods each. Both the teacher and social worker led the group in facilitating the discussions. Initially, the topics were introduced by the adults; however, it did not take long for the children to generate the topics themselves. They tended to state them as complaints: "My teacher expects me to do work I've never done before"; "All the kids look at me funny when I come into class at 10:30"; "I'm going to kick their ass if they don't let me play tomorrow." We usually restated the complaints in terms of "What do I do when . . . ?" Through the use of discussions and role playing, we tried to help them to examine alternative ways of solving problems, as well as the part they may have played in creating a situation that could have been avoided. Our goal was to help them to take a constructive and active role in confronting and resolving their problems. For example, in the situation where the child complained about the teacher's expectation to do unfamiliar work, we had the group members break up into teams and play the roles of child and teacher. Eventually, the child decided that he would tell his teacher that the work was new to him and suggest to her that he could get help from his center teacher if he could have some worksheets to show her. Once a decision was made to take a specific action, the child was expected to follow through and report back to the rap session what had happened. In this case, his public-school teacher agreed to give him the worksheets and also arranged for him to attend some early morning *help sessions* with her. She also arranged for him to work along with one of his classmates for extra practice.

An example of a universal problem faced by all the children had to do with the feelings they had about telling others that they had been at the center. This problem usually surfaced when they were asked such questions as "What school did you come from?" or "How come you only come here in the morning?" A typical answer was "None of your business!" But this response led, if not to a fight, to teasing based on speculation, such as "Mommy won't let her little boy come to school all day," or "I know, you go to a crazy kid's school." In the reflective atmosphere of our rap session, some children suggested more adaptive answers, using a friendly tone of voice, such as, "I go to a special school" and "I go to a private school." When these suggestions were tried out, they seemed to work, and if suggestions coming from the rap session worked, more credibility was given to this approach to problem solving. If they did not work, we tackled the problem again.

Assessing the Project. The transition program worked well because it was relevant. Problems and successes that were addressed were real. Memories of negative experiences in public schools could be diminished for the children, as well as their parents, through this intermediate step before returning to a neighborhood school placement.

The transition program described was changed as a result of both internal and external changes that took place simultaneously. First, as a result of staggering entry and termination times, we rarely had a single large group of children leaving the center at the same time. Next, public school policy no longer permitted youngsters living outside of the center's neighborhood school district to attend the school. Last, at around this same time, most of the school districts from which our children came began to take more responsibility for placing children from settings such as ours. Their own intake teams gather information on each child through testing, observations, and meetings with the treatment team and parents. Once an appropriate school and classroom are found, the child and center teacher visit the school, meet the principal, and sit in the classroom where he or she will be placed. Once a decision has been made for a child to leave the center, much of his or her concerns are dealt with as part of a group therapy experience with all the children in his or her classroom and/or during the child's individual psychotherapy meetings.

The Structure and Function of the Human Body

Introduction. It was not the children's driving curiosity and incessant questions that led to the development of a special curriculum on the human body. It was the four-letter words and other provocative language used to describe bodily parts and functions. It was the giggles, sly glances, and not-so-subtle innuendoes associated with boy–girl friendships. It was the obvious embarrassment and discomfort shown regarding the physiological changes that were taking place in the children who were approaching adolescence. It also came about as a result of a teacher's wish to have a clinician experience the difficulties and challenges of teaching a group of emotionally disturbed children. In other words, as a result of a myriad of very good reasons, only a few of which are mentioned here, a project was designed within the current science class aimed especially for a group of 10- to 12-year-old boys and girls and taught by two of our staff members, a teacher and a child psychiatrist. We called it The Structure and Function of the Human Body, in the belief that such a formal and somewhat antiseptic-sounding name would help, initially, to get the children to slip into the highly charged subject area without too much anxiety and aggression. The classes were held for 1 hour each day, 5 days a week, over a period of 3 months.

Sequence and Content. The planners believed that the sequence of the course was as important as the content, presenting what they deemed as the "less clinically relevant parts" at the beginning of the project and ending up with the material on human sexuality, working from top to bottom, so to speak. In carrying out the project, however, we learned that almost any part of the body could be clinically relevant to at least one child. For example, the brain touched off questions about being crazy and/or being retarded, and the heart about being loved and cared for. Children who wore glasses wanted to know what went wrong and could it be fixed. The ears concerned those children with reading problems who had trouble distinguishing word and letter sounds. Children who were poorly coordinated and chosen last for team athletics had some trouble regarding muscle functions. Not surprisingly, kidneys and bowels were a focus not only for enuretic and encopretic children but for the entire class. By the time the topic of the day was the sexual organs, the children had already safely dealt with a great many sensitive issues and felt able to explore this highly charged area with relative comfort, judging from the nature of their questions. Here are just a few examples: "How come I'm not a boy?" "Did it hurt when I came out?" "Do you have to be married to have a baby?" "Why do girls bleed?" "When can I do *it*?"

Activities and Discussions. Questions were always encouraged. Different approaches were used to supply the answers: Models were constructed and viewed, films and slides were shown, and encyclopedias and other books were consulted. The children were a fund of information, both correct and incorrect. Emphasis was placed on learning the scientific word for each body part and its function and noting that these new words were not used in the same way many of the old words were.

People's reactions to loaded words, family values, attitudes, and behavior were very much a part of the discussions as well. There were times during the course that information the children already had was discrepant from what we were teaching them. Some of these discrepancies were based on misinformation; others had to do with attitudes and values. Our discussions dispelled the misunderstandings and fostered respect for the differences in attitudes and values expressed.

Present Status. This special project continued for 4 years in its original format and at times included medical students who were on an elective rotation. Sections of the project were gradually integrated into the regular curriculum, with some modifications made in content and activities for the younger children.

The Movement Activity Reading Program

How Did It Come About? The Movement Activity Reading Program (MARP) was born out of teacher desperation and the admission that "hitting the books" described what the children and teachers were doing, literally, after a reading session.

For Whom Was It Meant? The initial group consisted of 10 children, 5 acting-out, four withdrawn, and one borderline psychotic child. Although the number of children varied over the life of the program, it never fell below 10. Ages ranged from 7 to 13, and the reading instructional levels spanned zero to low fourth-grade level. All the youngsters had negative attitudes toward books, teachers, school, peers, and self. There were four adults (one full-time and the others part-time) involved in one or more of the centers. The purposes of MARP were to channel aggression into learning, foster participation of withdrawn children, and encourage all of the children to engage constructively and actively in the reading process. In theoretical terms, we got our inspiration for this action learning model from Dewey and Piaget.

Of What Did It Consist? For 90 minutes each day, these children were engaged in *movement* activities within six centers, each with graded, sequential skill levels to meet each child's instructional needs. No child was forced to write or to read before he or she recognized the need to do so; the activities, however, were designed to elicit this need. Fifteen minutes were allotted for each center, but there was some flexibility within each center, based on need, attention span, and interest.

The first and sixth centers required total group participation; the other three were carried out with either a child alone or two to three children together. The fourth and fifth centers each started out as a solo activity, progressed to a small group, and eventually included the total group. This progression was dependent upon the children's ability to express themselves verbally. The sequencing of the centers was the same each day, and each is described briefly here.

Center 1: Body Awareness and Relaxation. This center was designed as a transition period from arrival and morning playground activities to the more sedentary activities in the classrooms. The activities were planned to help the children develop an awareness of their physical and mental state and how they could shift from a state of tension to one of relaxation and vice versa. The whole group engaged in structured movement and relaxation activities for 10 minutes. Directions were given orally and/or with large written cue cards. When the children first entered the room they were expected to lie down on the floor and breathe deeply and expel their breath slowly. Another favorite warmup activity was to think of themselves as rag dolls, starting with relaxing their heads and necks, and gradually relaxing each arm and hand, and finally each leg and foot. In order to increase their awareness of the difference between being tense and being relaxed, they would alternatively tense up and relax different parts of their bodies. The director and a child volunteer would check the children to see if they had been able to accomplish the tension and relaxation states. If not, the children having difficulty were given extra assistance and encouragement. As the children became familiar with the sequence of the directions, they took turns as directors until a new set of activities was introduced.

Center 2: Writing Stages. This center was aimed at helping the children to recognize, interpret, and use written symbols as a means of meeting their need to convey information to others. Each child progressed from game-oriented exercises in the early stages, to pencil-and-paper work exercises in the later stages. For example, letter sound, letter name, and/or word-recognition activities might be designed around the use of a large rubber floormat marked off in squares to be used with square rubber cards, a stamp and ink pad for table work, large cutout upper-and lower-case letters for tracing, and a typewriter. At times these were used individually, but wherever feasible, children worked in groups of two or three.

Center 3: Reading Stages. Through captivating props, activities, and pupil-and-teacher-made stories, the goal of this center was to encourage every child to become an active participant in learning and improving his or her reading skills. Puppets, plays, stories, and word games, mostly teacher made, were the activities around which the reading stages were designed. For example, the Movement Activity Reading Series was a collection of original stories by the teacher, some of which were present-ed on cards shaped to match the subject of the story (e.g., a dinosaur shape for *Dinosaur Bones* and a hammer shape for *Hammers Are for Hammering*). The stories that were written or selected were based on topics and themes of interest to the children. A series of detective stories were written that provided clues in the stories that would lead to another story card. In other words, the stories gave the children a reason for reading, involved movement, and were fun. The children could work alone or in pairs.

Center 4: Language and Concepts. The purposes of this center were to promote the development of language concepts, the ability to express these concepts clearly and accurately to others, and the opportunity to listen to and learn from others. There were two approaches used in this center, one that used the sense of touch, the other that focused on the ability to discriminate sounds. For the first a box called the Think Box was used. Items that could be described by the way they felt were placed in the box, one at a time. Such items as a key, measuring cup, apple, and thermometer were used. Each child felt the object that was concealed in the box. Then, all the children participated in asking questions about its characteristics, uses, and related properties. A "20 questions" format was used. When it appeared that nearly all the children knew its identity, the teacher would give the okay for the child to name the item. (For a fuller description of this activity, see Cooke & Parsons, 1969.)

For discriminating sounds, a tape recorder was used. Familiar sounds, such as a lawnmower, hair clipper, pencil sharpener, and running water, were recorded by the teacher and played. Again, using the 20-questions format, the child elaborated on the *when, where,* and *why* of the target sound until nearly all the children recognized it before it could be named.

Center 5: Listening and Problem Solving. The primary function of this center was to provide each child with the opportunity to identify with characters and situations similar to her or his own and to encourage a range of solutions to the conflicts the characters faced. It attempted to turn the stance of passive victimization into active mastery. A child was asked to listen carefully to a story read by the teacher and to comment on what was happening and say how he or she would deal with a similar conflict in his or her own life. After the children became comfortable relating to stories on an individual basis, this became a group activity that increased the spontaneity. The group also benefited from having at least several resolutions to conflicts in a story.

Center 6: Evaluation. This whole group activity was an attempt to help each child assess how a particular behavior contributed or detracted from his or her daily performance. The children had their own charts listing two or three behaviors on which each was working (e.g., day dreaming, temper tantrums, interrupting, and participating). They evaluated their own behavior first, and then the other children and teachers gave their opinions. The rating scale included 10 points, with 10 representing the best rating possible. The final rating was arrived at by group consensus and recorded by each child on his or her own bargraph. Initially, the teacher selected the behavior that the child needed to improve and recorded the rating that was arrived at first by the child and then by discussion and group consensus. However, as the children demonstrated their ability to look at their own behavior more realistically, they were given the responsibility of selecting behaviors on which to work and in recording their own ratings.

The Nuts and Bolts. In order to keep the program flowing smoothly, there had to be a great deal of team work involving the critiquing of lesson plans, the creating of highly motivational activities and materials, daily documentation of the children's progress in each of the centers, and daily, regularly scheduled meetings among the four adults responsible for the program. The daily plans for the centers, although completed in advance of the day they were to be used, were implemented with flexibility. Each adult had the opportunity to question the content or presentation of an activity and to suggest alternatives. Following its use with the children, notations were made in the margins of the daily lesson plans and incorporated later in the revisions made for the next group of children who would work through the centers.

There were endless opportunities to be creative; each adult's input was highly valued. It was this kind of teamwork that made the project uniquely exciting for all of us but especially for the graduate teacher trainees who had opportunities to be creative in developing new activities that soundly taught specific reading skills.

Outcome. The children demonstrated an increasing willingness to participate in the language activities with energy, concentration, and pleasure. They showed an increased willingness to participate in unfamiliar tasks and grew in their ability to assess their academic performance and behavior realistically. This was a significant change in both attitude and behavior. The teachers worked together cohesively, energetically, and enthusiastically. Creative abilities were unleashed and accompanied by a sense of comraderie, stimulation, and satisfaction. The MARP continued for a period of 3 years. When the teacher who had been its primary mover left for health reasons, MARP was reorganized and carried out within the more traditional structure of the four classrooms. Perhaps the most important concept transferred in this reorganization was that emotionally disturbed children could be motivated to participate actively in their own learning to their and their teacher's benefit.

Practicing the Three Rs: Letting the Chips Do the Talking

The Problem. After an intense morning program involving a range of positive and negative interactions between pupils and teachers as they struggled with academic subject matter and relationship problems, there was a need for some distancing among them. There was also a need for the children to practice their reading, spelling, and arithmetic skills and assume increased responsibility in their own learning. What was needed was a low-pressured, nonjudgmental, highly structured, and highly motivational project, one that would neutralize the interaction between the adult and child and was focused on success. A contingency-based reinforcement project, which was being carried out as part of an individualized tutoring program in the public schools by a colleague at the Medical Center* sounded as though it might be adaptable to an individualized group tutoring program. We arranged for several consultations with her and came up with what we believed to be the best elements of cross-age teaching and a contingency-based reinforcement project. The details of this project are described next.

The Solution

The Sessions. Individualized contingency-based reinforcement, skill-practice sessions were planned for each pupil four times a week, during the first hour following lunch. The sessions were organized in three 22-minute time segments. Groups of five to six children met in one of the classrooms that was set up with numbered tables, one table for each child. Poker chips, pencils, and spelling sheets were on the tables.

The Teachers. The teacher could be any staff member including a teacher, or it could be a child. The children coveted the teacher role; it implied competence and authority. Additionally, some students appeared to perform better with their peers than with adults. An effort was made, therefore, to assign a productive match of student and teacher.

*Bonnie W. Camp, PhD, MD, had developed a tutorial program for the Denver Public Schools using paraprofessionals in the teacher role. Dr. Camp is Professor of Pediatrics and Director of the John F. Kennedy Child Development Center at the University of Colorado Health Sciences Center.

The Expectations. As the children entered the project room, an over-sized chart by the door gave the following information next to each of their names: the table number where they would be working and the name of the person with whom they would be working for that day. They were expected to read this information and go directly to the table assigned. The children were also expected to pick up a designated arithmetic box, word cards, reading folder, and score sheet, and bring these materials with them to the table.

All the children were expected to begin each practice session at the same time on time. The loss of the full potential of chips that might be earned was the natural consequence of being late. Chips were not awarded for behaviors involving a value judgment by the teacher. Performance on the day's lesson was the focus.

The Lessons. Each child worked at his or her own level and progressed at his or her own speed from lessons designed in small sequential steps in each subject area. Practice levels were arrived at through the results of the Gilmore Oral Reading Test and through teacher-made tests in word–letter recognition, spelling, and arithmetic.

One teacher activated the timer for all of the children. Each child worked on clearly specified tasks with the teacher: 4 minutes on specific arithmetic facts, 5 minutes on oral and written spelling, and 5 minutes on reading skills. The remaining 8 minutes were taken up by recording the number of chips received at the end of each of the three time segments and the total chips received for that day at the end of the last practice segment. Counting and recording were done by the children when possible, thus giving additional practical exercises in arithmetic and writing.

Chip Values. Chip values remained constant across subject areas: two blue chips or four red chips were equivalent to 1 point. Each subject area had its own scoring format, however. In arithmetic, one blue chip was awarded for a correct answer on new material; a red chip was awarded for the review. New words could be studied for as long as the child desired. In spelling, review words were dictated first, and a child earned two blue chips for each correct word. One chip was given for orally spelling the word correctly. Next a child was expected to spell a list of words correctly by writing each word from dictation, a task that earned one blue chip for each word written correctly. If time was left, the child could write any of his or her words for one red chip each. Red chips were awarded for second attempts or for reviewing a lesson within the same time segment.

For most children, the reading lesson began with vocabulary cards worth one blue chip each. This was followed by a segment of reading the word in context, for which they could earn three blue chips for each paragraph. Finally, there were comprehension questions for one blue chip each. Beginning readers often worked on letter names and appropriate phonics and word-attack skills.

Corrections were made in a nonjudgmental fashion, primarily by showing a child the correct answer rather than by verbalizing it. The child then repeated the correct answer twice. There was a box to check that said, "Go on," if mastery was demonstrated, or another that said, "Hold," if a repeat of the same lesson was called for the next day.

Tallying the Points. A teacher and two children who were volunteers or selected at random, tallied the points at the end of the week. Students earning 150 points or more could spend these points on "priced" items (e.g., models; coloring, puzzle, or maze books; toy cars, hair ribbons, jacks, and playing cards) or on a highly valued activity (e.g., baking cookies with the center's cook; going on a trip to the park, neighborhood convenience store, public library, or record shop). Another popular activity was time in the Crafts Shop, making something out of wood, puppets, or simply using a hammer, nails, and paint to construct something original. Some children, usually the older ones, elected to save their points until they had 400 (the limit) and then go to a special store to purchase a more expensive item such as cassette tape or large model.

Evaluation. During the 3-year life of the project, the staff members believed that the outcome was both positive and negative. On the positive side, most of the children were able to work with a variety of people who were in the teacher role. Power struggles between adults and children appeared to decrease dramatically, accomplishing, in effect, the aim to neutralize those relationships. In addition, the children seemed to recognize that what they learned resulted from their own efforts. Furthermore, their views of themselves as academic failures seemed to shift as they experienced success and earned chips.

On the negative side, however, was the limited amount of skill and behavior that transferred to other parts of the program. When the children left the room, they left behind most of what they had learned of the three Rs and took with them the pleasure derived from trading in their chips for the item of their choice.

In critiquing the program, the staff members felt that they needed to focus more heavily on creating a learning environment where transfer of learning would occur. In attempting to utilize the positive aspects of the project and minimize the negative aspects, a somewhat less formally structured contingency-based reinforcement program was included in the morning educational program within the context of an integrated curriculum.

People-to-People Travel and Study Project

Introduction. Over the 5-week summer school period, 10 children between the ages of 10 and 13 years old participated in a human relations project that we called People-to-People. This project grew out of our belief that an important aspect of self-esteem develops from a strong sense of self, past and present, and of one's place in the universe. It was our impression, however, that the children we have seen at our day treatment center have either a distorted or weakened sense of both personal and family identity. Their knowledge about where they and their families come from, what they do, and what they like and dislike in the process of carrying out their lives is often incomplete and inaccurate. In addition, their understanding of their place in the community tends to be confused. In general, their sense of a continuous flow of history from past to present to future is almost nonexistent, and their view of the world as a dynamic, changing, living organism is lacking. The aim of the project, therefore, was to help these children to become aware of their roots and of their place in the community and to develop an appreciation for the richness within themselves and others and of the similarity and diversity among all people.

In the process of developing this awareness and appreciation, it was planned that the children would learn social, communication, recreational, and group-living skills. In addition, they would have the opportunity to apply the Three Rs in real-life situations. This was to be accomplished through thoughtfully designed, highly motivational activities involving a wide variety of media. The project was designed by three staff members: a teacher, a social worker, and a psychologist. Funds were obtained from two sources, the U.S. Office of Education Title IV-C funds through the Colorado Department of Education and from a private donor.

From the Known to the Unknown. During the first 2 weeks of the project, the children studied about themselves and their families by interviewing various family members and answering questions about themselves. The children represented their own personal history in a variety of formats, such as booklets with photographs or drawings, answering such questions as Who am I? Who do I live with? What are my favorite foods, cartoons, etc.? and What do I want to do when I grow up? Maps were used to locate cities, states, and countries where families came from or traveled through. Recipe books were compiled of favorite family recipes. A group profile was drawn, using this information to highlight the similarities and diversities of their characteristics and living situations. There were some concerns that the children who had experienced losses and other traumatic events would be unsettled by delving into their past. The adults working with the children were alerted to this possibility and attempted to structure and monitor the context within which the assignment was made and carried out. It was our impression over the course of time that the children were not adversely effected by these assignments.

During the next 3 weeks, the children used similar techniques for collecting and communicating information about their teachers and other adults at the center (Week 3), people in various walks of life in the neighborhood in which the center was located as well as in which the children lived (Week 4), and finally, people living in rural Colorado communities, both in the mountains and on the plains (Week 5). In effect, the project focused on what was most familiar to the children and moved, sequentially, to what was least familiar. At each new reach-out point, the children applied the knowledge and skills gained in the previous weeks, refining and adapting those skills to each new situation.

The Staff and Children Plan Together. The four adults who accompanied the children on the journey around Colorado included a classroom teacher, teacher aid, psychiatric social worker, and a graduate teacher trainee. The children were involved directly in the planning from the start. This process involved such decisions as clothing and equipment needed, menus for the 5 days, places to visit, and people to interview. The activities during the planning stage involved shopping, bookkeeping, packing, map reading, and letter writing. Job assignments were made for the 5 days as well. These jobs included setting up and breaking camp, cooking, making brief journal entries, map reading, interviewing, and photographing. There were very few discipline problems, a factor that we attributed to the children being so deeply involved and immersed in the events of each day.

A wide variety of skills were learned and some of them mastered, such as those involving social interactions (e.g., cooperation, communication, and problem solving) and day-to-day living (e.g., keeping accounts, map reading, and meal preparation). In addition, they learned first-hand about the way contemporary Native American Indians live in Colorado as compared to the past, the ins and outs of ski resorts and mining camps, the lives of the trappers, and of the wide range and beauty of Colorado's physical geography.

The End. The people who had initiated and carried out the program had moved to other positions and were no longer available to organize the project. Most critical, however, was the fact that there were no volunteers to take their place. Thus, what had been a very successful program faded into obscurity—at least until this description brought its existence to light once more.

ACKNOWLEDGMENTS

The development and implementation of the MARP project in 1974 was supported, in part, by a Teacher Award from the Colorado Department of Education ESEA funds.

The development and implementation of the People-to-People project in 1980 was supported in part by a Team Grant from the Colorado Department of Education, under the auspices of Title IV-C of the Educational Amendment Act (95-561).

REFERENCES

Camp, B. W., & Van Doorninck, W. J. (1971). Assessment of "motivated" reading therapy with elementary school children. *Behavior Therapy, 2,* 214–222.

Cooke, R. M., & Parsons, P. C. (1969). The listening class: An opportunity to advance skills of attending to, concentrating on, and utilizing auditory information in emotionally disturbed children. *Journal of Special Education, 2,* 329–336.

III

Administrative Issues

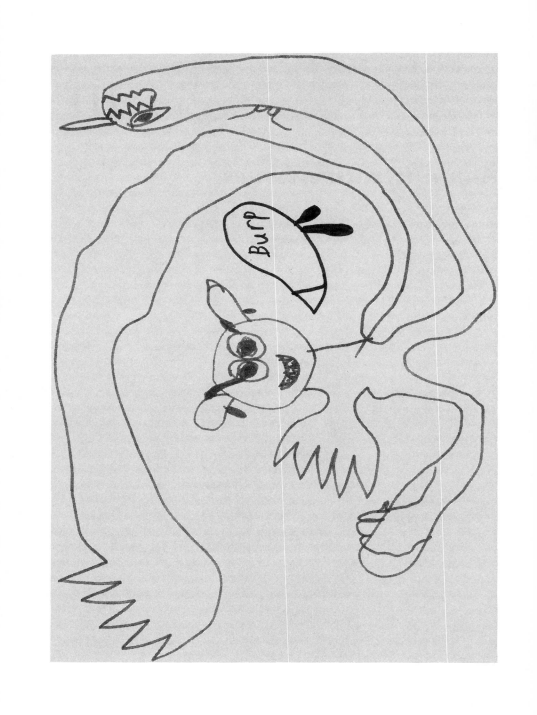

The very nature of a program built around multiple services to our children and their families within the context of a milieu makes divisions among them artificial. The reader will no doubt notice that there is much overlapping between and among the program components. Nevertheless, we felt obliged to identify the predominant focus within each of our chapters. Thus, although many administrative issues are touched upon in most of the chapters, we are left with only two chapters in this section, one on financing our program and the other on the implications of how several members of our treatment staff view their roles.

In Chapter 11, Gordon Farley reviews the current status of the complex mix of funding sources available for our day treatment program. Based on our own experience, he is careful to caution the reader that these sources are likely to disappear at any moment despite very good reasons for the continued support of day treatment. This caveat is amply documented and provides a strong rationale for flexibility, ingenuity, and perseverance in the face of serious odds.

Through individual semistructured interviews with six of our key staff members (three teachers, two social workers, and one child psychiatrist), Sara Zimet examines the personal and institutional attributes that may contribute to reducing the phenomenon of "burnout" that plagues mental health professionals in intense treatment settings such as ours. "Day Treatment Staff View Their Roles" (Chapter 12) contains very personal statements that communicate both a universal and a setting-specific message. It touches upon areas of concern that are applicable to all complex systems providing intensive mental health services and, therefore, deserves the reader's careful attention. Anyone working in settings similar to ours will recognize the issues, resolved and unresolved, discussed here.

11

Funding a Day Treatment Program

GORDON K. FARLEY

INTRODUCTION

In these times of changing patterns of referral, changing payor mixes, rapidly rising medical costs, changing demographic patterns, shrinking public funds, and increasing demands for service, the key to survival for a day treatment center is often sound financial management rather than providing high quality or effective treatment. Although these two possibilities are not mutually exclusive, neither do they automatically coexist. In the relatively short span of 10 years, our day treatment center has moved from the enviable position of being supported at a rate of about 95% from nonfee sources to being supported at a rate of about 80% from fee and contract for services sources. In other words, 10 years ago we were little concerned about billing and collections, whereas today we are obsessed with the everyday reality of finances. Financial matters permeate every discussion and clinical decision.

Despite the fact that day treatment facilities have been shown to have equal efficacy at a lower cost than do 24-hour-a-day inpatient settings (Gabel & Finn, 1986; Herz, Endicott, Spitzer, & Mesnikoff, 1971; Moscowitz, 1980; Zimet & Farley, 1985), children's day treatment facili-

GORDON K. FARLEY • The Day Care Center, Department of Psychiatry, University of Colorado Health Sciences Center, Denver, Colorado 80262.

ties have been underutilized and short lived all over the United States in recent years (Fink, Longabaugh, & Stout, 1978).

An important factor in our longevity and current financial stability is a full-time administrative officer. The responsibilities of this person include evaluating all patients referred for their ability to generate payment and assure collection from these sources. In our day treatment center, payment sources include the following:

1. Medicaid.
2. Contracts with social services departments.
3. Private health insurance carriers.
4. Out-of-pocket fees from patients.
5. The Authorized Revenue Base from public schools.
6. Excess costs contracts with public schools.
7. The State of Colorado budget appropriation.
8. The U.S. Department of Agriculture.

In addition to these traditional sources of revenue, we also obtain funds from other sources such as research grants, training and program support grants, and independent fund-raising efforts.

Each of the 11 sources listed are discussed in turn. In the final two sections of this chapter, the role of the finance committee in assisting families with health insurance matters is described.

MEDICAID

Our largest source of funding at the present time comes from Medicaid payments for services rendered. We now receive approximately $600,000 annually from Medicaid, and this represents about 70% of our total income from charges for our clinical services. In the State of Colorado, Medicaid pays for (a) approximately 80% of our daily charge of $165 per day, (b) 80% of our charge for two sessions of child psychotherapy per week, and (c) 80% of our charge for one session of parent therapy per week. Because of the availability of Medicaid reimbursements, we have been accepting more patients who are eligible for these funds. Naturally, we are deeply concerned that this important source of funding may suddenly be diminished. For example, limits may be set on length of treatment as has recently occurred for inpatient care. We feel the necessity of being poised to rapidly move from one funding source to another by seeking new sources of referral and changing our payor mix.

CONTRACTS WITH SOCIAL SERVICES DEPARTMENTS

At times we are able to negotiate contracts for long-term treatment of children with the respective County Department of Social Services. Lengths of contracts vary from 9 months to unstipulated treatment periods; however, all patients under such contracts require a periodic review to confirm continuing need for the level of care offered. The fees that we recover for the treatment that we provide have gradually increased until, at the present time, we receive $1,100 per month for a 12-month year. This represents only slightly more than one-quarter of the charge for services we provide. County departments of social services, however, vary in their willingness or ability to purchase day treatment from us. For example, they may disagree with our philosophy of treatment; they may wish to keep the money in their own county; or they may prefer to select a treatment center that offers reduced services at reduced cost.

THIRD-PARTY PAYERS

For medical insurance written in the State of Colorado, the benefit for day psychiatric hospitalization must be twice the length of the benefit for inpatient psychiatric hospitalization. Currently, the minimum benefit requires 45 days per year of inpatient hospitalization that transposes to a minimum of 90 days per year of day psychiatric treatment. In some cases, however, children's inpatient benefits have been arbitrarily reduced to an unspecified figure that is below that available to adults. Another threat to the formula stated is Diagnostically Related Groups (DRGs). Although DRGs are not yet enacted into law in Colorado, they are becoming more and more common for inpatient treatment in many states. The treatment provided by some hospitals for certain DRGs can be as brief as 10 days.

Many health insurance companies do not specify or announce day treatment as a benefit. In negotiation with them, however, it becomes clear that it is indeed a benefit. The importance of uncovering this information is obvious.

OUT-OF-POCKET PAYMENTS FROM PATIENTS

Some of our families have the resources to pay for a part of day treatment, and some have health insurance policies requiring a co-payment. With these families, we negotiate an agreed upon fee to be paid in addition to whatever else we recover in fees from other sources. These fees never completely compensate us for the total cost of the treatment we provide. They are set on the basis of the families' ability to pay, with due consideration given to their income and outstanding debts. This latter category includes medical expenses, which in many cases are quite high.

AUTHORIZED REVENUE BASE

In the State of Colorado, under Senate Bill 428, which was enacted into law during the 1981 session, our day hospital is entitled to bill the Colorado Department of Education for the state average per pupil operating cost for each child enrolled in our facility. This is known as the Authorized Revenue Base (ARB). Billing is done monthly on a full-time equivalent (FTE) basis. A child enrolled for an entire month is considered one FTE. The amount of revenue designated for 1990 for each FTE is $3,760. For our population of 24 children, this resource generates $90,240 for the year. Agencies that operate a 12-month school program bill each month and receive one-twelfth of the state average per pupil operating revenue amount for each FTE each month. Agencies that operate a 9-month program are expected to bill on a 9-month basis and will be entitled to one-ninth of the state average.

EXCESS COSTS

In the State of Colorado, when there are additional costs associated with the education of an emotionally/behaviorally disturbed or learning-disabled child in a non-public-school setting, the public school's Department of Special Services will agree to pay the excess educational costs, as approved by the State Board of Education. They expect to review with our facility the child's continued need for treatment placement at least every 6 months. The excess cost rate is approved by the State Board of Education for each facility for all children identified as handicapped and who have an Individual Education Plan (IEP) in place. For our facility, the excess cost rate is $17.32 per child per day with an indirect cost rate of $8.73 per day. However, it is not required that the indirect cost rate be paid, and to date we have not been able to negotiate such payment. Whereas the rate for excess costs is set by the State Department of

Education, the individual contracts on each child are negotiated with that child's home school district. Excess costs currently generate approximately $35,000 to $40,000 per year. This figure is expected to increase as more contracts are obtained. Currently, 9 of our 24 children are funded for excess costs. This has been a very important source of revenue in the last two years.

Whether or not we are successful in obtaining these funds appears to depend heavily on our relationships with the individual school districts. A school district must agree that the child has an educational handicap, that this handicap cannot be properly remediated in a regular classroom setting, and that they do not have the educational resources to provide the necessary remediation in their district.

STATE OF COLORADO APPROPRIATION

The State of Colorado makes an annual appropriation to the University of Colorado Health Sciences Center. A portion of that appropriation is applied to the operating expenses of the Department of Psychiatry, which then determines, on a year-to-year basis, how much money will be allocated for the operating expenses of our treatment program. The total funding from the State of Colorado appropriation to our program last year was $240,000.

RESEARCH FUNDING FROM EXTERNAL SOURCES

The majority of the research and program evaluation conducted at the Day Care Center has been funded from our general expense budget. Since 1975, a considerable portion has been funded from external sources. For example, most recently, we were awarded a small grant from the National Institute of Mental Health (NIMH) to aid us in our data analysis. In the past, we have had several small grants from our own institution's fluid research fund and from the Developmental Psychobiology Research Group, a research consortium endowed by the Grant Foundation and housed at the University of Colorado Health Sciences Center. These grants, totaling approximately $40,000, have been used to start up new projects, to complete projects when funds have been exhausted, and to initiate and complete whole studies. A review of the research carried out with the day treatment children as subjects is summarized in a chapter by Zimet and Farley later in this book.

TRAINING GRANTS AND PROGRAM SUPPORT GRANTS

During the 27 years of its functioning, training grants and program support grants have been sought and received on many occasions from state and federal agencies primarily through the efforts of the Day Care Center Director and the Day Care Center Director of Research and Program Evaluation. The training funds received from NIMH have been used to support both faculty and staff positions.

Training Grants

Day treatment of children played an important part in the most recently funded child psychiatry training grant from 1986 to 1989. We received approximately $160,000 over the 3 years. Day treatment has always received strong emphasis in our training programs, and trainees in adult psychiatry, child psychiatry, psychology, and social work have always had some components of day treatment experience, varying from small to very large. During the 3-year period, the training grant supported some salaries in our day treatment program. The emphasis of the grant was on the treatment of underserved populations. In our setting, training in day psychiatric treatment has been recognized as a critical and mandatory part of training in child psychiatry. The necessity for mandatory training in child day treatment has not been recognized either in our setting or nationally for social workers, psychologists, or adult psychiatrists. This situation is intimately linked with the lack of federal funding to provide this type of training.

Program Support Grants

We have obtained several grants from federal and state agencies that have offered us technical assistance in the adoption of validated programs and support for library programs and special motivational learning programs. Examples of the adoption of validated programs are the Colorado Department of Education Friends Project developed by Richard Boersma (1982), and aspects of the Developmental Therapy Program developed by Wood (1986). For more details about these and other projects, see the chapter by Parsons and Imhoff describing special projects and the chapter in Volume 2 by Swan, Wood, and Jordan on building a statewide program.

Support also was obtained from the State Department of Education for our children's library and for our motivational learning programs, one dealing with reading and the other dealing with social studies. In addition, we obtained matching funds to buy discounted paperback books for the children's home libraries from the national Reading Is Fundamental project.

Financial assistance toward making necessary repairs and replacing worn-out furniture and curtains was received from the Helen K. and Arthur E. Johnson Foundation. In order to resupply necessary toys, puppets, blocks, cabinets, trucks, and games for our children and our therapy rooms, we obtained a grant from the Faculty Wives Association of the University of Colorado Health Sciences Center. During the last 10 years we have received approximately $33,000.

THE U.S. DEPARTMENT OF AGRICULTURE

As a local educational authority, we are eligible for funding from the U.S. Department of Agriculture for the school lunch program. Depending on the socioeconomic mix of our population, we get a set amount for each lunch and snack we serve to our children. At times, we also get commodities at very low prices or at no cost. Our total payments from the Department of Agriculture amounted to $6,500 in 1989.

FUND-RAISING ACTIVITIES

In the last 4 years, fund raising from donors has become increasingly important. Under the direction of our administrative officer, we have had bake sales, book sales, children's art sales, concerts, holiday dances, rummage sales, garage sales, and other fund-raising activities. Through the fund-raising activities, we have established a fund known as the Child Resource Fund, which has a number of different purposes such as providing children in our program with extra activities that they would not otherwise be able to participate in, providing research funds, and providing funds for materials and supplies. To this date, we have raised approximately $10,000 from these activities.

THE FINANCE COMMITTEE

Our center's Finance Committee is made up of our assistant director, head teacher, administrative officer, and intake director. The charge of this committee is to negotiate contracts with social services departments, departments of education, Medicaid, and third party payers. In actual practice, these contracts are negotiated by our administrative officer with the consultation and approval of other finance committee members and the director. Another responsibility of the finance committee is negotiating fees with families and assuring their ability to pay for services, either directly or from other resources. The finance committee meets regularly with the administrative-intake committee, and the membership of the committees overlaps to a significant extent.

ACTING AS AN INSURANCE COUNSELOR FOR PATIENTS

Often, families who apply for treatment at the Day Care Center have woefully insufficient medical insurance. That insurance is particularly likely to be deficient in psychiatric coverage. Most of these families have children who have received treatment in at least two or more mental health facilities. In addition, many of these children are likely to be at risk for future psychiatric treatment needs. Therefore, we feel that it is important to inform the parents of potential mental health and physical health insurance needs. At times, we are able to assist families in obtaining adequate medical insurance, sometimes supplemented by Medicaid or Social Security Insurance. At other times, we are able to uncover insurance benefits that families did not know existed. This is done through direct negotiations between our administrative officer and the insurance carrier.

SUMMARY AND CONCLUSIONS

Our program is funded from a complex mixture of sources. Some sources fund patient care, others fund research, and still others fund extra projects and building refurbishing. These funding sources are in a constant state of change, as old ones disappear and new ones appear briefly only to vanish. Keeping a program operating requires an ability to rapidly adapt to changing funding sources and requirements.

REFERENCES

Boersma, R. (1982). *The "Friends" project.* Steamboat Springs, CO: Northwest Colorado B.O.C.S.

Fink, E. B., Longabaugh, R., & Stout, R. (1978). The paradoxical underutilization of partial hospitalization. *American Journal of Psychiatry, 135,* 713–716.

Gabel, S., & Finn, M. (1986). Outcome in children's day-treatment programs: Review of the literature and recommendations for future research. *International Journal of Partial Hospitalization, 3,* 261–271.

Herz, M. I., Endicott, J., Spitzer, R. L., & Mesnikoff, A. (1971). Day versus inpatient hospitalization: A controlled study. *American Journal of Psychiatry, 127,* 1371–1382.

Moscowitz, I. R. (1980). The effectiveness of day hospital treatment: A review. *Journal of Community Psychology, 8,* 155–164.

Wood, M. M. (1986). *Developmental therapy in the classroom* (2nd ed.). Austin, TX: Pro-ed.

Zimet, S. G., & Farley, G. K. (1985). Day treatment for children in the United States. *Journal of the American Academy of Child Psychiatry, 24,* 732–738.

12

Day Treatment Staff View Their Roles

SARA GOODMAN ZIMET

INTRODUCTION

"Burnout" is a concept frequently associated with professionals who succumb to stress from working with troubled children and their families. In some centers, it has resulted in a turnover of up to 50% of their staff members. We have experienced very little turnover among our educators and clinicians. The current professional staff has been working at the center from between 7 and 27 years and appears to be able to handle the stresses associated with providing intense habilitative and rehabilitative services to a sometimes reluctant, intractable, and intransigent group of children and parents. What are the forces that help to buffer these stresses and reduce the likelihood of staff turnover? Some of the answers may lie within the structure of the program itself, which, at its best, brings professionals together in a cooperative egalitarian effort to fulfill a mission. Other answers are likely to reside in personal characteristics and in particular attitudes and values that also function to cushion stress.

In an attempt to identify both institutional and personal stress-buffering characteristics, a representative sample of professionals on our staff, three of our five teachers, two of our three social work clinicians,

---

SARA GOODMAN ZIMET • The Day Care Center, Department of Psychiatry, University of Colorado Health Sciences Center, Denver, Colorado 80262.

and our director, a child psychiatrist, participated in individual semi-structured interviews. The questions they were asked centered around what they considered to be the core of their work, how it differed from working with children and families in other settings, what personal characteristics made them suitable for their job, what they liked most and liked least about their work, what they considered to be the most difficult part of their work, and what they would like to change in their present work setting if they could. In the paragraphs that follow, the responses to these questions are presented verbatim, first those of the teachers, then those of the social workers, and finally, those of the director. Although we believe that their words speak for themselves, this writer could not resist closing this chapter with a discussion of some of the more obvious forces revealed by the interviewees' answers.

INTERVIEWS WITH TEACHERS

Chris Wilcox

These kids need so much support and attention. In addition to having serious emotional problems, most of them have learning problems. I feel a great responsibility to provide them with appropriate and interesting learning experiences. One of my strengths as a teacher is that I am willing to make the extra effort needed to motivate them, to stimulate interest and excitement about learning. I especially enjoy teaching them new things using a variety of media. When they get interested in learning, they get out of themselves and stop thinking about their troubles. I try to be primarily positive with the children, praising their efforts, and trying not to emphasize the negative behaviors. Working with these children is very challenging.

It is easy to get discouraged because everything you do seems to get undone so quickly. One minute they are on-task; the next, they are elsewhere. They are so easily distracted by noises in the hallway or in the playground or by their own thoughts. Another difficulty is that, as their teacher, I am frequently made the target of all their anger and frustration. As their teacher, however, I need to understand where that anger is coming from, and I try to be there for them all of the time, psychologically and physically. Teaching these children is a high-intensity experience, especially in my work with the younger children.

There are two behaviors that get my goat: whining and overt aggression. When a child whines, I label it as not acceptable and ask the child to tell me, in a more appropriate way, what he or she wants. If the whining continues, I give the child a time-out to think of a better way to tell me what they need or want. When two children are fighting or one child is throwing things and out of control, I thank the other children for staying out of it, and I call for assistance from either my teaching assistant or from another staff person (see the chapter by Farley on Standby), whoever is readily available. My goal is to calm the child or children down as quickly as possible and keep the rest of the children composed and safe.

One of the hardest parts of working here is trying to leave work behind me at the end of the day. I have gone through a lot of stages on this issue. For my own mental health, I need to do this. When I first began working here, I felt that nothing was going right. I couldn't make things better for the children. They didn't seem to be changing in ways that I had expected, and I worried about them to the point of losing sleep. I felt overwhelmed by all of it. I think it was important for me to realize that I could survive these bad times of feeling like a failure. I gradually realized that it wasn't up to me only, and that perhaps other parts of the program weren't always working as they should be. The therapists frequently would come late or cancel a session and not let the child know. Standby was often backed up and not available when I needed it. There were undercurrents among the staff that were not worked out. I realized that some things I could control while other things I could not. I tried to take a more philosophical, more pragmatic attitude toward my work. This has helped.

The best part of working at this center is the people I work with. We have a very resourceful staff who have the willingness and wherewithal to get things done. The worst parts are the number of people coming and going—trainees and visitors—and the need to train and orient people to the same material over and over again.

I would like to see more staff interaction with the children through-out the week so that the classroom is not an isolated area of treatment. I would also like to have a larger classroom so that I could separate the activity areas better.

I feel that it is very important to keep in touch with the parents daily by sending a note home with each child that shows how the child did that day in school. While the emphasis is on the positive behaviors shown, the absence of positive comments in some areas lets the parents know that there are still areas their child is working on. I also make it a point to call a parent when the child is absent from school, to find out why she or he is out and when we can expect the child to return. I like to make either

phone contact or send a newsletter home at least once a week with each
parent to keep them informed of our classroom activities.

Willard Edwards

Respect for one another—that is really important. At the start of the
year, I set the structure and pace of the classroom and establish who is in
charge. As the students show that they are able to take some responsibility for their own behavior, the structure and pace change.

Establishing rapport and trust with children comes naturally to me.
Maybe they respond so well to me because of my size, and they feel that I
can protect them. But sometimes I wonder if it is because they are afraid
of me, being so big and strong. Humor is another tool I use with them
when it feels appropriate. I never talk down to them; I literally bend to
their level and make eye contact with them. I want them to know that I
respect them and I expect them to respect me.

My major goal is to help them to behave more appropriately so that
they will get ahead in public school, so that they will fit in and not stand
out like a sore thumb. I want them to learn how to give their teachers
some pleasure and that, in turn, the teachers will respond positively to
them, will help them to get ahead. In my own experience as a student, I
saw some really bad kids, or turned-off kids, turn around when they had
a teacher who was interested in them. This is the kind of teacher I want
to be. I want the children to begin to feel good about themselves, to see
that they are capable and can succeed in some areas. I expect them to
work hard and do their best—to show me that they are trying.

The children take out on me what has happened elsewhere in their
lives. They also know which button to push to get my goat. They get my
goat when they try to find excuses for what they have done by telling me
that so-and-so does it, too. They get me going when they are not willing
to accept responsibility for their own actions.

I think it is very important for teachers to experience a child on a
one-to-one basis just as it is for the children's therapists to experience
children in a group. This could be done through classroom observation
or from first-hand interactions.

Next to working with the children, the "A-number-1" job of the
teacher is to get to know the parents well, to develop a relationship with
them and try to engage them in helping their child. The home and the
school should be working together. I think we should have parent
groups once a month. If the parents won't come to us, then we should go
to them. Contacting them by phone once a week to let them know how
their child is doing, with an emphasis on the positive, is crucial.

Patricia Mulligan

I like the intensity, the total involvement required in working with children in this kind of setting. I like the focus on learning a lot about each child and planning a program to suit them individually and as a group member. Yes, the children are very disturbed, very demanding, and very challenging, but I like it.

There is a fine line between dealing with children's individual needs and the needs of the group. I sometimes think of it as a balancing act. I have set up a program of positive reinforcement for individual and group behavior. The children are rated for each 10-minute time block throughout the day. This way I am assured that the children are receiving feedback on both negative and positive behaviors.

When the children are out of control in a very aggressive manner and the atmosphere becomes emotionally charged, I become very concerned for the safety of the children. I respond very quickly to these situations by removing the aggressive child or children from the room. I let them know that this behavior is not acceptable, that they need to calm down and gain control of themselves before they can come back to the classroom. Sometimes a time-out will suffice; other times, I will call for a "Standby" to supervise the time-out or to calm the child or children in some other way. If the child runs away, I will call a Standby for help. My teaching assistant does help in individual behavior management problems as well.

I am especially good at teaching the individual children at their own level and pace. The range of abilities in my group is enormous. I first identify the positive qualities in each one of them—their strengths. I provide a great deal of structure; I follow through on my expectations, encouraging each of them to take responsibility for their own behavior; I help them to make friends; I offer them opportunities to develop a sense of being a group.

The children's first reaction to any new learning situation seems to be, "I don't want to do it, it's dumb, it's stupid." It is up to the teacher to set the stage for learning, to motivate the children to want to learn. Then it is up to the children to act and, eventually, to become responsible for learning.

It is vital that all parts of the program communicate, coordinate, and integrate. This should be done through the team. I like working as a member of a multidisciplinary team, where treatment decisions are arrived at by the participation of all members, where there is respect for everyone's opinion. The concept is great, but it doesn't always happen that way. It depends on the team leader. The psychotherapists have the edge. When there is a conflict among the team members there needs to be a process established which will deal with the problem. Healing among team members is essential and in the best interest of the children and their parents.

I don't feel that the therapists place a very high value on the child's educational experience here. For the child whose life is chaotic at home, the classroom provides reasonable expectations and a great deal of structure. The child is able to find success here. This is an area of his life over which he can gain some control, some competence. It can provide the child with a way out of an environment which he cannot control. Coming to school is a child's occupation.

I try to reach out to all the families. I feel it is important to establish frequent communication with them. I extend a welcoming hand to the children's parents by phoning them each week, not just when there is a problem. I keep in closer touch with them when the child is home sick. Sometimes I find out very important information in this way—that the family is planning to move, that they are separating, or that someone is moving in to live with them. If they wish to set up a behavior modification program at home, I will help them to do this. Each day I send a note home with every child. Sometimes I will write a note and request an answer. Some mothers will stop by and chat when they pick their child up, but most of the children are brought to and from the center by a transportation service.

I would like to have a more spacious classroom so that I can carry out a greater variety of activities and projects. I only have space for desks. We also should have a separate observation area for parents, therapists, and visitors. I would like to have videotaping of my interactions with the children. I think that kind of feedback is very powerful and very useful. The supervision for teachers should be more consistent as well.

INTERVIEWS WITH SOCIAL WORKERS

Abe Tenorio

My job consists of three areas: clinical, administrative, and training. I am heavily involved in doing treatment—both individual and groups, with both children and families. As a result, I work closely with many of our treatment teams. I don't have any preferences for one kind of psychotherapy over another. I like all aspects of my clinical work. I have two child therapy groups; each meets once a week. The teacher and teacher assistant in each group act as my co-therapists. I like working together with other staff members like this. I only do groups with classes that agree to it. If a teacher does not want us in, we stay out, and this happens sometimes. I think it has something to do with "territoriality," whether the teacher is able to share his or her classroom group with others. Working with the children in their classroom groups helps me to get a better picture of what they might be like in their own family groups. If I am seeing the parents of the children in the group, it gives me an appreciation for the parents' dilemma, and it helps me to understand how interactions with others influences the children's behavior. My cotherapists and I meet to review our work whenever our schedules allow— approximately once every 3 weeks. We do give some assignments to the children. For example, George's task was to take responsibility for his behavior by not getting into fights with the other children for the next week. The individual group members provided him with feedback during the week, and George and the group members reported on what had occurred at the next group therapy session.

I feel that individual therapy also is very important. There are many issues that you cannot deal with in a group because of the need for confidentiality. In addition, many of our children are from families where secrets are prevalent. One form of therapy may work with some kids but not with others. I do individual child and parent therapy and family work as well. There are times when I feel it is appropriate to have family meetings without the child present.

I believe that as a child's therapist, it is very important to work closely with the parents' therapist, and this is our center's policy. The team provides the mechanism for doing this. Many of the child fellows and other trainees who do child psychotherapy choose not to do this. I think it's because they prefer to work alone, and some don't realize what our ground rules are about working on a team.

As I work with a family, I try to determine what approaches work best. I believe that it is important for me to be flexible. Since finances have become critical around here, I have been concerned that my personal code of ethics will be challenged; I may have to decide between what is best for the patient versus what is best for the center. For example, we can no longer take any patients who do not have Medicaid, who cannot pay anything, or who have poor insurance coverage. So far, there really has not been a big problem because there are many children who need our help who can pay for it.

Medicaid right now is our best payment resource. While we are not compensated for all the group therapy that we do, we feel it is a very valuable treatment modality. As a matter of fact, I feel that all our classrooms should have group therapy, and we are trying to figure out how this can be done with our present staff.

One of the things that I like about my job is being able to see changes in some parents and kids. I think individual and family therapy does have an impact on how they function. But I also realize that the changes might not last, that they only may be temporary. I guess the reality is that some patients do change and some don't. Some go back and forth while they are here in treatment and also after they leave. I get a feel for who will make it and who will not. Eric, for example, I think we helped him not to be so crazy. His parents, though, are pathetic, so needy and dependent. We couldn't get them to move. In therapy, we worked toward the parents separating. Now, they are getting a divorce and I think that's a good thing because it may help to break the self-destructive cycle in their relationship. I also hope that they will become more aware of their children's needs. Couples therapy didn't work so it had to be done individually. My approach with them was very directive and concrete. I guess that with some families, I am left with a feeling of hopelessness. My goal is for them to achieve a better level of functioning.

I like teaching the social work interns. We have had good and bad interns. It's not an easy job, but I enjoy the relationships I develop with them; I enjoy being a mentor.

I think that I am relaxed and accepting of most people, and people in turn feel comfortable with me. Some people are suspicious and difficult, but in general, people are receptive to what I have to say. I don't usually come on with guns and pushing things down people's throats, and I think this characteristic of mine helps me to be effective in my work at our center.

I take work home with me, not just the worry about how the families are progressing but work that I wasn't able to finish up before 5 o'clock, such as phone calls and tying up loose ends. I do carry with me my concern about filling up slots in our program because I know that we need to do this in order to keep the program going. I also think about the fragile cases—those who are suicide risks. I try not to be preoccupied by my work or to let it affect my family life. But I am not ever completely free of it unless I leave town and immerse myself in unrelated activities.

Before coming to work here, I had 9 years at a state mental hospital. I worked on an adult outpatient community team, an inpatient adolescent locked unit, and an adult inpatient unit where I was a team leader. I find more gratification here. I like the size of this unit, and I like dealing with other agencies and systems. I like working with our staff. I feel that I am knowledgeable, and some people respect that. Of course there are some who don't, but most do. There are differences of opinion, of philosophy, and among personalities, so things don't always go smoothly. In general, though, the staff is a very cohesive group and we get along well, talking and working together. I have worked with a lot more difficult groups of people than those on our staff, and those experiences make working here look and feel pretty good to me.

This is my wish list: (a) no hassles from our department; (b) less of an overbearing financial situation; (c) teachers' assistants all day rather than half a day; (d) a substitute teacher; (e) a clinical psychologist to do testing and treatment; and (f) one more full-time social worker.

Caroline Corkey

There are three roles that I perform: teaching, clinical, and administrative. Many of the things that I do within each of these roles I created for myself because role definitions evolve informally in our center. For example, as a faculty member in the Department of Psychiatry, I have never had formal teaching responsibilities assigned to me. The teaching that I do in the introductory course in psychiatry to the medical students happened when I was asked by the coordinator of that course if I would like to lead a postlecture discussion group and I agreed to do it. Another example of this informality is my supervision of one of my colleagues at the center, who requested me to do this for him. Well, I am a senior member here so it makes sense for me to help out. I guess what I am trying to say is that when there is a need and if it matches my interest, I do it, with or without recognition.

As a part-time person, there are very few perks, and I guess that is why I look for things that I like to do to make up for the lack of salary increases and other forms of recognition.

Teaching at the center involves the supervision of one of the social work staff and of two to three of the trainees from Smith College School of Social Work. This requires approximately 2 hours per week per supervisee, plus the time involved in reading process notes and writing evaluations. My teaching also involves organizing the center's orientation program for all of the social work trainees from both Smith College and the University of Denver. The orientation covers all aspects of our center's program and takes 6 hours over 4 days to complete every September.

My administrative activities include being a team leader on six teams and coordinating our Standby program (see the chapter by Farley where this program is described). I also serve on several *ad hoc* committees each year, frequently as the chairperson, like the one that drew up the policy on our postlunch rehash meetings and the other that organized the pot luck dinner for staff and parents twice a year (see the Zimet and Schultz chapter on our food program where this is described).

My clinical work takes up most of my time. I am either the parent or child therapist for four families now (this fluctuates between two and four), and I run a short-term group therapy session once a week for 3 months for those children who are between psychotherapists (the trainees have left and the new ones have not arrived). In addition, I see one medical, nursing, or dental student in psychotherapy as my *pro bono* contribution to the Health Sciences Center.

The best part about working at the Day Care Center is the opportunity to work over a long period of time with the patients. It gives me the opportunity to develop an understanding of their lives and their troubles—to gather a lot of information and to develop a close rapport. I am able to make use of this information for planning interventions which, hopefully, will result in making a difference in their lives. I believe that the children are able to change despite the fact that their lives are disruptive and chaotic. I believe that the children are resilient and that I can help them to meet the demands of the stage of development they may be experiencing, by improving their self-esteem and their relationships with others—children and adults. I feel that I can help them to cope with the here-and-now, and that perhaps they will have a model for coping effectively later in their lives. Here at the Day Care Center, I think it is possible to interrupt the revolving door syndrome that is common in inpatient settings and decrease the separation patterns by treating the child and the family in a stable setting over long term.

The complexity of the referrals we receive is interesting and challenging. They usually have multiple diagnoses. They are difficult to treat—much more so than those I saw in the emergency room and the ones I now see in my private practice.

This leads me to the bad part about working here. The families are very difficult to work with, and bringing about change is hard to achieve. Most of the families are chaotic; character disorder among parents is common; and there is a resistance to getting help. At least the parents agree that the child should be here and that is a big thing, an important first step.

I do see myself as a flexible person, and I've had a great deal of professional experience with a great variety of people in a variety of settings. I am good at working with a lot of different kinds of people. I know how to shift from short to long term, and I know when something is an emergency. You have to start where people are, and I seem to be able to do this. I seem to have a certain humility about this work and recognize the contributions people make at all levels—from aides to teachers to different disciplines among mental health professionals.

I realize that no system as complex as ours is perfect and that problem areas will arise regularly. What we need, however, is an effective way of dealing with these inevitabilities. We have a strong, dedicated, loyal staff of professionals who are able to deal effectively with a very difficult patient population. Every day we help our patients work out their problems, either individually or within their family structure. For some reason, however, we are not able to work on the problems that beset us as a staff, problems that arise both from within the milieu and from outside it. We'd probably all agree that the problem was there but then make every effort to forget it and get on with the work at hand. That may work for a while, but as problems build they begin to be expressed in ways that undermine the effectiveness of the milieu. I guess the item at the top of my wish list is that we find a better way to deal with our problems than the one we are currently using.

INTERVIEW WITH A CHILD PSYCHIATRIST

Gordon Farley

I consider the survival of this day hospital program to be my primary goal—the survival of a program that provides high quality and effective treatment to children and their families. A secondary goal of my work is to investigate the effectiveness of that treatment by studying the population being treated. I became an academic child psychiatrist 23 years ago in order to treat patients, to educate medical students, residents, and others training to be mental health professionals, and to do some scholarly work. When I became the director of this center, I also expected to be concerned to some extent about finances and administration. At the present time, concern about finances and administration is in first, second, and third place, and patient care, teaching, and scholarly/research are all tied for last place.

One of the central differences about working here as opposed to working in other settings with children is the public nature of the work. To some degree, this is a "fishbowl" setting. All staff members' work is observable by all other staff members. This is both a pleasure and a problem in that one gets both positive and negative feedback whether one asks for it or not.

In order to keep in touch with ongoing clinical activity, I have felt that I should be involved directly with patient care in a number of ways. For example, about one-half of our children receive psychoactive medication at some time during their stay with us. I review and monitor these medications, and, unless the child therapist is a physician, I prescribe the medications for the children. I frequently discuss the medication with the parents of the child, and I meet with the treatment team for consultation when medication is being considered. In addition, I conduct the case reviews—those of patients during intake and over the course of treatment. I am a team leader of 2 of our 23 treatment teams; I eat lunch with the children once or twice a week; I am on call for Standby up to 3 hours each week (please see the chapter on Standby); I supervise the children one morning each week as they arrive at the center; and I go to the camp for the full 5 days each year both as the camp physician and as a supervisor of a group of children (please see the Mulligan chapter describing our camp program).

I believe that I have several personal qualities that make me suitable for my job as director. I have an evenness of character and a calming and quieting influence that I can bring to bear during times of crisis. I have tremendous respect for the unique contributions of staff members, and I hope that this respect comes across to them. I try to listen to staff members' complaints about working conditions, and I try to improve them if at all possible. I also try to support their personal growth and professional development when it means moving to a position of greater responsibility and better compensation. In general, I see myself as setting an example for working hard, caring about the careers of those with whom I work, and listening to their concerns and wishes.

What I like the most about my work is the relationships with the children, families, and my co-workers. What I like least are the tension-filled and conflictual relationships between me and the people with whom I work and among the people with whom I work. Human relationships are both difficult and rewarding, and it is natural that in a close-knit program such as ours, many conflicts would revolve around the issues of role, territory, authority, and control. Many staff members view themselves as quite willing to relinquish control, and other staff members as overly eager to establish control.

It is well known that disputes among staff members trickle down and adversely affect the care of patients (Jones, 1953; Stanton & Schwartz, 1954). Festering, hidden, internecine warfare can destroy a program. I see resolution of these conflicts as part of my job as the director. My intent, therefore, is to address these disagreements before they affect patient care.

First of all, I expect that staff members will put aside internal conflicts, unresolved personal issues, personal dislikes for other staff members, and theoretical/philosophical disputes, and work toward providing the best treatment they can. There are several forums where problem areas are discussed. For example, we have staff meetings twice a week, and when there is no set agenda, items of personal concern may be brought up for group discussion. At other times, I am available to meet with staff members to discuss problems with them privately, if they prefer. My office is in the center's building, on a highly trafficked corridor close to the center's entrance and classrooms. Unless I am seeing a patient or preparing for a lecture, my door is open, and I am ready to talk.

Staff members frequently come to my office complaining that another staff member is not doing his or her job, is rude and insensitive, is domineering and overstepping the bounds of his or her role, or is just a malicious, nasty, disagreeable person. As a first step, I will ask them to take their complaint directly to the alleged offender but urge them, before doing this, to look at their own part in the conflict. This last suggestion is usually met with accusations that I am nonsupportive and blind to the saliency of their side of the dispute. At times, I may offer personal observations regarding my view of the conflict, its possible causes, and potential resolutions. But I have found that these views usually are not greeted with enthusiasm. I have also stated my willingness to hear the complainant's view of my role in contributing to and perpetuating the conflict; this offer is usually warmly received. Negative observations about my administrative style are tolerated for a suitable (to me) period of time.

A strategy that I sometimes employ when staff members complain that we are not working effectively with a certain type of child, parent, or staff problem is to assign them to an *ad hoc* committee to consider the problem. We have had committees on research, parent work, group therapy, case assignment, child abuse policy, the integrated curriculum, crisis interventions, camp, and intake. These committees have brought disparate ideas together, and this has often resulted in effective solutions.

When it seems appropriate, I have offered to meet jointly with staff members who are in conflict with each other. Sometimes there is the shared feeling that face-to-face meetings, even with me present, would be of no help; other times, the offer is accepted or even demanded, and sometimes a resolution is reached. However, when all possibilities have been exhausted, I will ask the parties in the dispute to live and work in a polite, tolerant, and professional way with their co-worker(s) for the good of the treatment program. In a few instances, one of the combatants has left our center to work elsewhere.

In recent years, one cause for a great deal of stress among staff members has been the need for budget cuts. This has had a direct effect on staff layoffs and the elimination of valued program components. It seems to me that a striking parallel exists between the model for learned helplessness (Seligman, 1975) and the everyday realities of working in a setting that is a small-treatment cog in a large institutional wheel. Despite our best efforts, we are often unable to avoid the punishments of budget cuts, space loss, nonpayment of benefits, and personnel changes. My response is to try to demonstrate that we do have control over some of the important contingencies of our everyday lives, particularly those regarding the treatment of our children.

If it were possible, I would like to have institutional relief from the financial pressures, so that decisions about treatment could be made on the grounds of clinical judgment rather than economic necessity (please see my chapter on funding). In addition, I would prefer an atmosphere in which staff members would put aside their personal animosities, rivalries, and wishes for dominance, and work for the good of the children and families.

DISCUSSION

The primary focus of this chapter has been to identify some of the personal and institutional stress-buffering characteristics that appear to contribute to the low staff turnover at our center. Several characteristics seem to emerge consistently from across the interviewees' answers, whereas others appear to be uniquely associated with an individual. In general, teachers, social workers, and the director expressed genuine feelings of caring and respect for the children and their families. They were optimistic in their belief that change is possible and that what each of them does makes a difference in the children's and families' lives. Yet, this optimism is tempered by their grasp of the reality that bringing about change is more often than not a frustratingly slow and variable process. Although believing that they each possess the skills necessary to do their job effectively, they also valued the work of their colleagues and of the treatment-team structure. In support of this structure, sustaining good interpersonal relationships among staff members was seen as crucial.

Some paradoxes emerged as well. Two examples come to mind: First, in spite of the high value placed on good relationships among staff members, a consistent theme throughout the interviews is the presence of interstaff conflicts and the difficulties in resolving them; and second, although each interviewee expresses a high regard for his or her colleagues, most feel unappreciated and try to find satisfaction in other aspects of their work.

The use of defense mechanisms, such as projection and denial, also appears as a way of dealing with frustrating situations associated with one's role. As mental health professionals, it is important to be able to differentiate when these mechanisms facilitate and when they interfere with carrying out one's role effectively.

There appeared to be great care exerted in monitoring the carryover of work-related issues to other settings. In effect, there seemed to be an ability to bring to bear a great many personal resources that could effectively cushion the stress of working with this population of troubled and troublesome children and their parents.

Program attributes also appear to contribute to mitigating the effect of stress. There appears to be strong evidence that our treatment milieu consists of a supportive network of professionals working well together, *most of the time,* toward a common goal. In addition, the informal policies of the system appear to allow for a great deal of latitude in carrying out one's role and for finding intrinsic sources of job satisfaction.

Although the individual interviews point up the strengths within our system and within the people who work in that system, they also indicate undercurrents of concern. It is not surprising to find problems in treatment settings as complex and demanding as ours. Accepting them as inevitable and addressing them as they arise in various forums, such as staff meetings, problem-solving retreats, and individual supervisory sessions has proven constructive in the past. This approach speaks to an administrative structure that is willing to be responsive to the undercurrents and intervene in ways that are beneficial.

CONCLUSION

There appears to be a great deal of emphasis in the organization/administration literature today on managing the stress endemic in one's workplace. Stress management, in fact, has become a by-word associated with the prevention of burnout. In this chapter, an attempt has been made to identify personal and system characteristics that prevent and buffer stress within our day treatment setting. Although the personal characteristics of a staff contribute to this process, having a responsive structure within the program is essential as well. Both forces interact to bring about the desirable effects.

REFERENCES

Jones, M. (1953). *The therapeutic community: A new treatment method in psychiatry.* New York: Basic Books.
Seligman, M. E. P. (1975). *Helplessness.* San Francisco: W. H. Freeman.
Stanton, A. H., & Schwartz, M. S. (1954). *The mental hospital.* New York: Basic Books.

IV

Research and Program Evaluation

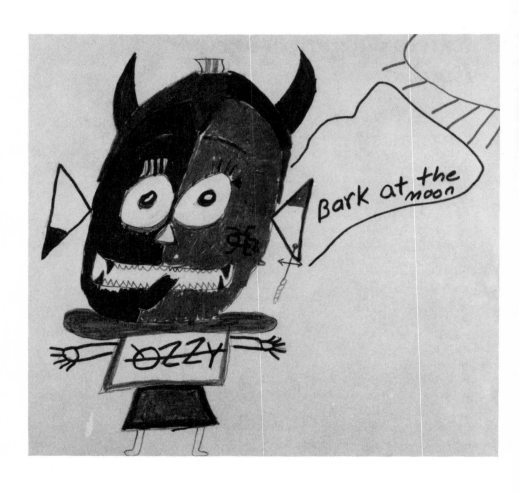

Quality assurance and therapeutic efficacy have been goals of our day treatment program since 1973. For this reason, we established and implemented a comprehensive data base and carried out research on various aspects of our treatment program. In this final part of Volume 1, the reader will find three chapters describing these efforts. In Chapter 13, Sara Zimet, Gordon Farley, and Nanci Avitable, our data base manager and educational test administrator, provide the reader with a thorough rationale and methodology for putting a data base into place in a day treatment setting. The authors contend that a data base contributes to clinical decision making, sets the stage for program evaluation, and provides a rich resource for testing hypotheses. The end result is improved clinical practice. Although this chapter strongly advocates the virtues of establishing a data base, it also acknowledges the difficulties that are likely to develop among staff members who differ in their views as to its value. We are both forewarned and forearmed by this exhaustive presentation.

In order to exemplify the richness that is inherent in a day treatment setting for those seeking to carry out research, Sara Zimet and Gordon Farley review the many studies they have carried out since 1973. In Chapter 14, "The Day Treatment Program as a Research Setting: A Review of Our Research," we are given much food for thought. The menu consists of follow-up studies, predictive studies, studies of competence and self-esteem, of achievement in reading, spelling, and arithmetic, of intelligence testing, and of hearing and auditory discrimination—14 studies in all. The authors transport the reader through the purpose, methods, and results of each of the studies and the connections between and among them. Each inquiry represents what appears to be a logical development toward the next investigation or series of investigations. Clearly there is much more work to be done, both in carrying out new research and in replicating what Zimet and Farley have found with other children and in other settings.

Finally, in Chapter 15, Caroline Corkey, a social worker, and Sara Zimet present us with a complete description of a follow-up study of adults between the ages of 18 and 25 years of age who were treated in our day hospital when they were children. The measure of adjustment in young adulthood was their current relationships with family and friends. The personal characteristics that might have contributed to the outcome were also examined. Although the difficulties associated with clinical research are discussed, the care taken to overcome many of these difficulties is impressive. The results make good clinical sense and should provide encouragement to other investigators eager to pursue clinical questions arising in complex settings such as ours.

13

Establishing a Comprehensive Data Base in a Day Treatment Program for Children

SARA GOODMAN ZIMET, GORDON K. FARLEY, and NANCI AVITABLE

INTRODUCTION

Although it seems self-evident that a uniform data base is useful in a clinical setting, this is, in fact, a rare event. To the best of our knowledge, few day treatment centers have made this a priority. In 1973, 12 years following the opening of our center, we set ourselves this goal of establishing a comprehensive data base. Our decision coincided with the increasing pressures to document the effectiveness of our treatment program. These pressures came from insurance carriers, consumers, and legislative and other governmental bodies allocating scarce mental health service funds. In the text that follows, the nuts and bolts of establishing a comprehensive data base are described and discussed with special attention given to both technical and human factors.

This chapter is reprinted from "Establishing a Comprehensive Data Base in a Day-Treatment Program for Children," by S. G. Zimet, G. K. Farley, and N. Avitable, 1987, *International Journal of Partial Hospitalization, 4,* 1–15. Copyright © 1987 by Plenum Publishing Corporation. Reprinted by permission.

SARA GOODMAN ZIMET and GORDON K. FARLEY • The Day Care Center, Department of Psychiatry, University of Colorado Health Sciences Center, Denver, Colorado 80262.   NANCI AVITABLE • 2833 South Wabash Circle, Denver, Colorado 80231.

HUMAN FACTORS

The idea of developing a uniform data base on each family origi-nated at the administrative level. As is the case with all important deci-sions, the idea was discussed at length with the entire day treatment staff and agreement was reached that an educational psychologist should be hired to provide the leadership for this new endeavor. Subsequently, such a person was added to the staff.

Although the usual procedures leading to staff consensus had been carried out, all members of the staff were not enthusiastic regarding this project. In retrospect, their reticence might be traced to one or more of the following reasons:

1. There was no need to change what appeared to be an adequate format for keeping records. We experienced this attitude at a time when our department was trying to shift from a narrative style of therapists' notes to a more structured problem-oriented one. The majority of our planning committee was pleased by this shift because it believed that this new approach to record keeping made it possible to document the treat-ment process with quantifiable data, whereas the old narrative approach did not.

2. The energy and staff resources should have gone to another part of the program, such as increasing administrative support in order to reduce the clinical work load. For example, some people felt that it would have been more judicious to hire a business manager rather than a data manager. If we had done this, we would have freed up a clinician to share more of the clinical work load.

3. It was threatening. The concepts of program evaluation and research may have conjured up a lot of negative feelings, such as "now they are going to find out what a terrible job I'm doing," rather than some positive ones, such as "now they are going to find out what a good job I'm doing." In reality, of course, both of these possibilities were likely. For example, in a recent research project, we taped clinicians doing crisis interventions with children over a 4-month period. The purpose of this project was to identify the components of this crisis intervention ap-proach that led to satisfactory resolutions. What we found was that five of the six interventions with unsatisfactory resolutions had been done by the same clinician. This clinician had asked for supervision of other work that was being done. Through diplomatic negotiations, supervision was provided that covered a broader spectrum of clinical activities. If this situation had been dealt with less diplomatically, we could have heightened the threat component of staff participation in research ac-tivities and increased the possibility of sabotage.

4. The traditional tensions that exist in a university setting between staff and faculty may have contributed to uncooperativeness. Staff members may have felt that the establishment of a data base is a faculty-serving endeavor, where their hard work provides faculty with the necessary stepping stones for promotion and does not serve nonfaculty staff any valid purpose.

5. There was a lack of understanding regarding the contribution that the systematic collection of data makes toward improving clinical practice.

6. Feelings of intimidation were generated at the prospect of learning about a new discipline or body of knowledge.

Whatever the reason, a lack of enthusiasm may be expressed in somewhat passive ways by delaying decisions, or more actively by delaying implementation of decisions, or by refusing outright to participate in the agreed-upon plan. Because of the destructive implications of these behaviors for effectively carrying out a milieu-oriented treatment program, we decided to include all the staff at each step of the way, from the initial planning stage to the implementation and maintenance stage. We hoped, in effect, to reduce staff resistance by increasing ownership of the project. We did this by organizing a steering committee, six people in all, composed of one person representing each discipline and/or treatment component of the program under the leadership of the educational psychologist (S.Z.), six people in all.

ROLE OF THE DATA BASE

The Steering Committee's first task was to define the role of a data base for our clinical setting. We reasoned that one well-defined data base could fill several partially separate and partially overlapping but always synergistic purposes: clinical decision making, program evaluation, and research. Each of these purposes, the processes associated with them, and the consequence of their interactions with each other are illustrated in Figure 1.

The three purposes served by the data base are listed across the top of the diagram. Each is seen as being related to the other two, and all are seen as contributing to improving clinical practice (listed at the bottom of the diagram). In the columns under each purpose is a list of the processes involved in fulfilling it. All three share some processes in common (e.g., generating hypotheses, treatment planning, and obtaining outside funding), although the focus may differ somewhat. Other processes re-

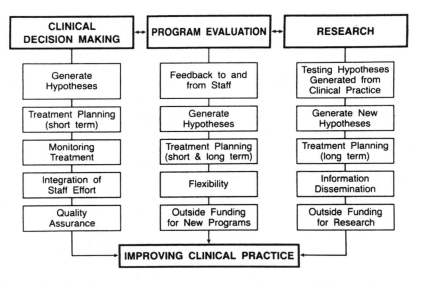

Figure 1. Relationship among purposes, processes, and outcome of the use of a comprehensive data base.

main unique to the specific purpose they serve (e.g., quality assurance, flexibility, and information dissemination).

Clinical Decision Making

Although treatment decisions are made on a daily basis in working with the children and their families, there are seven critical points at which these decisions take on particular importance:

1. When the parents and the child first contact the center.
2. When the intake evaluation has been completed.
3. When the initial planning is done for treatment recommendations.
4. When treatment progress is reviewed.
5. When terminating treatment becomes a consideration.
6. When planning for the transition to another setting.
7. When deciding to terminate outpatient treatment.

The following are some examples of how our data base has helped in the clinical decision making process:

Example 1. A 10-year-old boy who had been diagnosed as having a conduct disorder (undersocialized aggressive) was behaving very well in our school program. He was very compliant and cooperative, and he was making reasonable academic progress. There appeared to be a discrepancy, however, among his father's view of his affective state and the views held by other significant adults in his life. His teacher noted that he episodically appeared sad and depressed in school; his psychotherapist reported that he expressed thoughts of suicide; and his mother said that he cried inconsolably at times for no apparent reason. On the other hand, his father denied vehemently that his son was depressed because things were so much better in the family. As a result of the father's authority in the family, both parents refused to consider the possibility of giving the child antidepressant medication. The family's treatment team decided to obtain school and home behavior checklists (Achenbach & Edelbrock, 1983, 1986) from the teacher and parents and compare the scores with those obtained at the time the child entered the program 6 months earlier. The resulting scores showed that, although the child's aggressive and delinquent behaviors had decreased, his depressed behaviors had increased significantly, placing him above the 99th percentile. When these findings were shared with the parents, both father and mother agreed to a 3-week trial on an appropriate tricyclic antidepressant. After the 3 weeks, there was a marked reduction reported in the depressive symptoms in all three settings.

Example 2. Jeff, an 11-year-old boy who was bright, athletic, and good looking, had a persistent negative view of himself. This self-view was confirmed by his score on the Perceived Competence Scale for Children (Harter, 1978). On this test, Jeff was in what we called the "disparager category," the lowest classification in physical, social, and cognitive competence and in general self-worth (Zimet & Farley, 1985, 1987). We brought these low scores to the attention of his classroom teacher, his psychotherapist, and his parents and suggested that improved self-esteem be a primary focus of therapeutic and environmental work.

Example 3. A 10-year-old girl had been treated in our program for nearly 3 years. She had made considerable gains in nearly every area of development, but her parents felt that she was not ready to return to a public school setting. The parents had difficulty in recognizing the changes that had been made, possibly as a reaction to the move to another setting and fears of the future. As a part of the regular end-of-treatment data collection, we obtained the behavior checklists, the achievement test, the competence and self-esteem assessment, and the intelligence test. Significant gains were found in almost all areas tapped by the tests, and in her teacher's and parents' perceptions of her. When this information was shared with the family, it helped to reorient their view and calm their apprehensions about their child's return to a regular school setting.

Program Evaluation

Program evaluation is concerned with both short- and long-term planning. It involves an ongoing examination of every aspect of the day treatment program. Policies may be revised, communication patterns may be streamlined, and staffing needs may be reviewed and updated. For example, when the Steering Committee had determined what demographic information was important to collect about the child and family when they entered and left our program, it had an impact on the intake and transition procedures. Responsibilities had to be assigned and redefined and intake and transition packets prepared to facilitate the process. In another example, there was some dissatisfaction among a large number of our staff regarding how reports of suspected child abuse were being handled. Two of our staff members had attended special meetings dealing with various aspects of abuse and neglect. They were asked to draft a policy manual for our use, drawing upon already existing documents provided by social services and other local and national agencies. This was done, reviewed by our staff, revised, and finally incorporated into our procedures handbook.

The extent to which the results of program evaluation affect the basic characteristics of the treatment program needs to be carefully documented, particularly when planning to carry out efficacy research. If the program dramatically changes, then dates marking the time when the changes took place define the population to be examined.

Research

Research is seen as affecting long-term planning. It takes several years to accumulate a large enough group of subjects to examine some of the ideas generated from clinical practice and program evaluation. In addition, from the time a study is designed to the time it is completed, 1 or more years may elapse. Thus the impact of research on treatment planning and on program evaluation normally occurs at some future point. This impact does not happen automatically but requires a conscious effort to implement.

Because clinical decision making is done over the period of time during which the patient is in treatment, we see this as involving short-term planning and as being concerned primarily with immediate issues. Following the completion of the termination process, clinical decisions are no longer likely to be made and, therefore, no further data are collected for that purpose. This is not the case, however, for program evaluation and research. After the conclusion of treatment, the overlap is between these latter two purposes. Figure 2 illustrates this overlap.

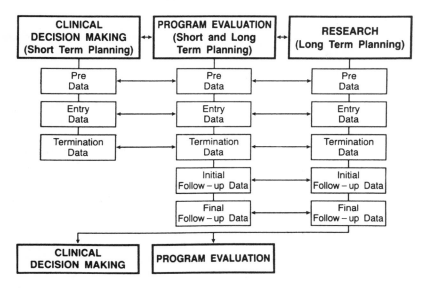

Figure 2. Data collection times for each of the three purposes of a comprehensive data base.

SELECTING APPROPRIATE MEASURES

The next task the data base committee tackled was the selection of measures that would serve the multiple purposes of making clinical decisions, evaluating the program, and carrying out research. We began by agreeing on the seven criteria that the measures were expected to meet. Each of these is stated next:

1. They should serve the three purposes mentioned before: clinical decision making, program evaluation, and research.
2. They should tap a variety of areas of the children's lives such as academic and intellectual performance, behavior at school and at home, peer relationships, self-esteem, auditory and visual discrimination abilities, and parents' psychological health.
3. They should be representative of several perspectives of the child's behavior, such as the child's, the parents' or caretakers', and the teacher's.
4. They should be psychometrically sound, demonstrating good validity and reliability.
5. They should be standardized on relatively large populations in order to provide normative data with whom to compare our day treatment children.

6. They should be relatively brief to administer.
7. They should be quantifiable in order to permit comparisons across subjects and among variables.

Because of limits on our spending, our steering committee had difficult decisions to make regarding the time periods for data collection and which instruments were to be collected at the designated time periods. Although we would have liked to include a midtreatment collection time, for practical reasons we could not, but plan to at some future date. We also would have preferred to collect the full battery of tests at the initial and final follow-up times. This, too, was not feasible. Thus we selected only those measures that did not require us to be present and that could be mailed to and from the informant. We made one exception by including the achievement test at the final follow-up.

The measurements selected, the person from whom the data is collected, and the timetable for collecting the data are shown in Table 1. Many of the measures are collected directly from the child, one from the child's teacher, several from the parents about the child, and one from the parents about themselves.

Table 1. A Comprehensive Data Base: Measures, Informants, and Collection Times

Measure	Collection times				
	Pre[a]	Entry[a]	Term[a]	IF-U[a]	FF-U[a]
Child Behavior Checklist (Achenbach & Edelbrock, 1983)		Parents	X	X	X
Teachers Form of the Child Behavior Checklist (Achenbach & Edelbrock, 1986)	Former teacher	DCC teacher	DCC teacher	Current teacher	X
Adult Symptom Checklist-90-R (Derogatis, 1983)		Parents	X	X	X
Wide Range Achievement Test (Jastak & Jastak, 1978)		Child	X		X
Intelligence Test for Children, Revised (Wechsler, 1974)		Child	X		
Auditory Discrimination Test (Wepman, 1973)		Child	X		
Perceived Competence Scale for Children (Harter, 1978)		Child	X		
Developmental Questionnaire		Parents			
Demographic Information		Parents	DCC staff		

[a]Pre = during evaluation; entry = in treatment program; term = end of treatment; IF-U = initial follow-up 3–6 months after term; FF-U = final follow-up 1 year after IF-U.

WHO DOES THE WORK?

Carrying out the day-to-day work of collecting data and maintaining our data base involves all of our staff members some of the time and two of our staff most of the time. These two are directly responsible for overseeing the data collection efforts for all three purposes. They administer tests to the children, collect checklists from teachers and parents, score tests and checklists, update the data base, prepare entry and termination reports from the test and checklist data, design and carry out research, analyze data, disseminate the results of research, and/or generate funds to support research.

CLINICAL CHART DATA

In addition to the data described in Table 1, information about each child prior to admission and during treatment at our center is kept in a loose-leaf notebook referred to as the child's clinical chart. This information is listed in Table 2 along with its source and the times it is collected and recorded. It includes documentation of past events that are likely to have affected the patients' present status as well as new data that de-

Table 2. Data Kept in Each Child's Clinical Chart, Informant, and Entry Times

| | Time periods | |
Data	Entry	Termination
Signed letters of informed consent	Parents	X
Past reports and records	Agencies	
Current physical exam report	Physician	
Mediation chart	Therapist	X
Entry and termination test reports	Psychologist	X
Intake summary	Team leader	
Developmental rating form (Wood, 1986)	Teacher[a]	
School progress notes	Teacher[a]	
Team notes	Team leader[a]	
Lunch supervisor notes	Staff[a]	
Staff meeting minutes	Adm. sec.[a]	
Case conference minutes	Adm. sec.[a]	
Therapy notes	Therapist[a]	
Transition report and recommendations		Team leader
Patient termination summary		Therapist

[a]Indicates records are kept throughout treatment period.

scribes their current functioning. Treatment process notes fall into this last category. They are derived from various parts of the program. In addition to providing a broad picture of what is happening in the milieu, they enrich the meaning of the objective data listed in Table 1. Thus, all pertinent information used primarily at the critical decision-making points described earlier is located in one place and is easily accessible to the child's team and to other interested staff members. These records are typed, filed, and kept up-to-date by the center's support staff.

OUR DATA MANAGEMENT SYSTEM

We employ both a manual and an automated management system to store, process, and communicate our data. Where financial constraints exist, however, a manual-only data management system may be thought of as a first step in developing a rationale for a more sophisticated automated system to be installed at some later date. Both systems are described in detail next.

Manual-Only Management System

In a manual-only information management system, data may be filed in two ways. The two methods we have used are illustrated in Figures 3 and 4.

As seen in Figure 3, the data collected in Table 1 may be filed by time periods for each child. Each time period bears a different color code. All data collected at the pre- and entry-collection times are color coded green and stored in the green section of the file drawer. When a child completes day treatment, the folder is color coded orange and moved to the orange section of the file drawer. The orange file includes the termination data and indicates that the child is moving towards the initial follow-up data collection stage. After the initial follow-up is completed, the folder is color coded blue and moved to the blue section of the file drawer for the last stage of data collection, the final follow-up stage. The child's folder is then color coded red and moved to the red section of the file drawer for future reference. These folders serve as the backup structure of our automated management system. The files within each color-coded section are kept in alphabetical order.

The second way data from Table 1 may be filed is to assign a file folder for each piece of quantifiable data, such as the Child Behavior Checklist or the Wide Range Achievement Test, for each of the five time periods. This approach is illustrated in Figure 4. There are pretest files,

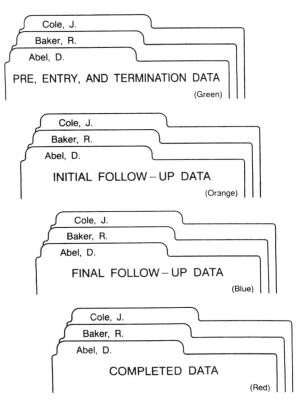

Figure 3. A manual-only data management filing system: color coded by time periods and filed alphabetically by children's names within time periods.

entry test files, termination test files, initial follow-up test files, and final follow-up test files. Within each of these file folders the tests may be filed alphabetically by the child's name or chronologically by the child's chart identification number.

Automated Management System

An automated management system may use a microcomputer only, a mainframe computer only, or a combination of both. For a small data base, an in-house microcomputer is probably the most cost-effective management system. Such a system also insures confidentiality. In choosing the machine to be used, one needs to know about its storage

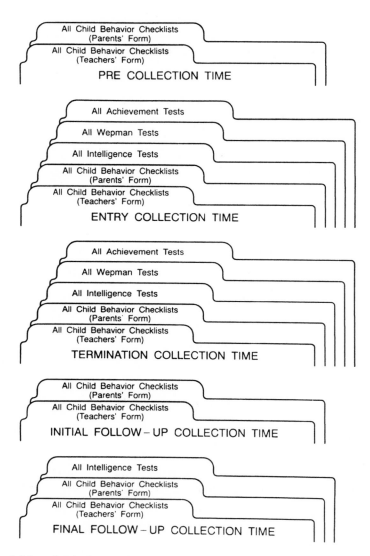

Figure 4. Manual-only data management filing system: each measure in a separate file for each time period and each measure filed alphabetically by the children's names or chronologically by their identification numbers.

capacity and available software. Most of the software designed for micro-computers is business oriented and may not provide the user with the ability to obtain desired or necessary statistical reports. Recently, pro-grams have been written to administer and/or score some of the more popular psychological test instruments. We have also written some of our own (N.A.). However, such programs have been designed to run only on the most commonly used equipment (e.g., IBM and Apple II PCs).

When using microcomputer systems, one must remember to fre-quently backup the data that are being entered. This is done by making more than one copy of a file. The floppy disks that are used for this purpose must be handled with care. Because of their size and shape they can easily be bent and abused in a number of ways, such as attaching them to paper with paper clips or storing them in a place where the sun's rays hit them. Any of these abuses are guaranteed to permanently wipe out the data on the disk. In addition, disks should be stored in a dust-free, magnetic-free, cool place. Finally, it is advised that backup disks be kept in a separate storage area from where the originals are kept.

A management information system that makes use of a mainframe computer will be more expensive. If cost is not a factor, use of a main-frame offers the following advantages over a microcomputer: (a) data storage capacity is greater; (b) data can be manipulated and/or trans-formed with greater ease; (c) a greater variety of data analysis packages are available, such as SPSS (the Statistical Package for Social Sciences) (SPSS, Inc., 1983); and (d) data can be transmitted and received intra-state, interstate, and internationally by magnetic tapes or by one of the electronic mail networks.

Unless one is fortunate enough to be able to afford an in-house mainframe, there could be a problem with confidentiality. This is partic-ularly true when using a commercial time-sharing service. On the other hand, the advantage of an outside service is the availability of technical personnel that one might not be able to employ directly. Also, all large commercial services regularly backup data stored on their machines and some retain these backups for a number of years.

Keep in mind that the computerization of a data base gives one the ability to produce more information than can ever be used meaningfully. Data to be examined need to be selected judiciously. This can be done by stating well-defined hypotheses about the areas and variables you wish to explore.

We began with a manual-only data information system. As we accu-mulated enough subjects to warrant group analyses, we moved to a mainframe computer. Further along, as microcomputers became more affordable and the software available promised to increase our ability to

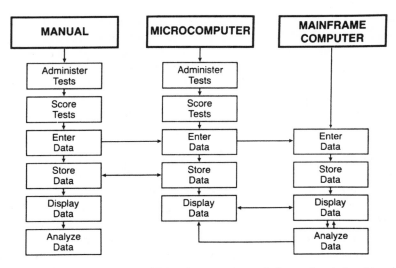

Figure 5. Summary of three data management systems used alone or in relationship to one another.

process and use the data more efficiently, we combined the three systems. Figure 5 summarizes the three systems described and demonstrates how the manual-only system relates to and intersects with an automated management system using both a microcomputer and/or a mainframe computer.

Communication between the micro- and mainframe computers is carried out by telephone through the use of a modem. This enables us to access the SPSS package (SPSS, Inc., 1983), which provides suitable programs for analyzing our data. Along the way, of course, we hired people with the specialized training to be able to use the technology of our data management system efficiently and effectively. We were able to develop and grow in this manner because our center director (G.F.) had made a major commitment to this endeavor. His commitment, in conjunction with publications based on our data base (Zimet & Farley, 1985, 1986, 1987; Zimet, Farley, & Dahlem, 1984, 1985; Zimet *et al.*, 1980), provided a strong rationale for the consistent support we received from our department chairman for further development.

ONGOING WORK

Although the members of our steering committee have changed over the years, the committee continues to meet to design new collection forms, revise old ones, make decisions on the addition or deletion of standardized tests and checklists, and review plans for the implementation of data collection for special projects. Many of these special projects have been supported by agencies outside our treatment center (e.g., our Medical School, the State of Colorado, and the Federal Government) and have involved additional subjects and data collection at times other than those specified on Table 1 (Blager, Zimet, & Farley, 1983; Corkey & Zimet, 1987; Farley & Zimet, 1987a,b; Jackson *et al.*, 1979).

Recently we received research funds from the National Institute of Mental Health to further analyze the data we have been collecting since 1973. We intend to carry out a series of studies with the following aims: (a) to identify and describe behaviors observed by parents and teachers at the four time periods shown in Table 1; (b) to compare subjects showing different profiles of change in severity of disturbance during specified time periods and to identify developmental and demographic variables that may be associated with these profiles; (c) to compare the school behaviors of children in day treatment with normal children in regular unmodified public school classrooms, with children referred to an outpatient clinic, and with children referred for inpatient treatment; (d) to determine whether emotionally disturbed children at the beginning of day treatment show patterns of cognitive functioning that distinguish them diagnostically from each other, from normal children, and from children in inpatient treatment; (e) to determine whether children at the beginning of day treatment show different patterns of cognitive functioning than at the conclusion of day treatment; (f) to contrast demographic and developmental characteristics of children in day treatment notably deficient in academic performance with those only moderately deficient and those functioning at expected academic levels; (g) to identify changes in academic performance over time; and (h) to contrast demographic and developmental characteristics of children who perceive themselves as being of little worth with those who are within the normal range and those who are grandiose in their self-views over time. The hypotheses for this project were developed primarily from the results of a pilot study published in 1980 (Zimet *et al.*, 1980) as well as from subsequent studies carried out by the first two authors and their colleagues.

CONCLUSION

Establishing a comprehensive database that meets the multiple needs of a clinical setting has made it possible for us to learn a great deal about the children we see in day treatment. It has also given us the opportunity to ask many more questions and to attempt to find the answers to these questions. Through this process of examining data collected systematically over the years, we hope to be able to discover which children make what kinds of specific gains in a specific setting, with a particular kind of intervention. The more settings in which these studies are carried out, the better able we will be to increase substantially our knowledge and understanding of children needing and receiving day psychiatric treatment.

REFERENCES

Achenbach, T. M., & Edelbrock, C. (1983). *Manual for the Child Behavior Checklist and revised Behavior Profile.* New York: Queen City Printers, Inc.

Achenbach, T. M., & Edelbrock, C. (1986). *Manual for the Teacher's Report Form and the teacher version of the Child Behavior Profile.* Burlington: University of Vermont, Department of Psychiatry.

American Psychiatric Association. (1987). *Statistical manual of mental disorders* (3rd ed. rev.). Washington, DC: American Psychiatric Association.

Blager, F. B., Zimet, S. G., & Farley, G. K. (1983). Auditory discrimination abilities of emotionally disturbed children in day psychiatric treatment: A replication study. *Journal of Auditory Research, 22,* 77–82.

Corkey, C. L., & Zimet, S. G. (1987). Relationships with family and friends in young adulthood: A follow-up of children treated in a day hospital. *International Journal of Partial Hospitalization, 4,* 97–115.

Derogatis, L. R. (1983). *SCL-90: Administration, scoring, and procedures manual* (2nd ed.). Towson, MD: Clinical Psychometric Research.

Farley, G. K., & Zimet, S. G. (1987a). *Cortisol excretion of emotionally disturbed children in relationship to stress, anxiety, and competence.* Unpublished paper, University of Colorado Health Sciences Center, Denver, CO.

Farley, G. K., & Zimet, S. G. (1987b). Can a five-minute verbal sample predict the response to day psychiatric treatment? *International Journal of Partial Hospitalization, 4,* 189–198.

Harter, S. (1978). *The Perceived Competence Scale for Children manual: Form O.* Denver: University of Denver.

Jackson, A. M., Farley, G. K., Zimet, S. G., & Gottman, J. M. (1979). Optimizing the WISC-R performance of low and high impulsive emotionally disturbed children. *Journal of Learning Disabilities, 12,* 56–59.

Jastak, J. F., & Jastak, S. (1978). *The Wide Range Achievement Test manual.* Wilmington, DE: Jastak Associates, Inc.

SPSS, Inc. (1983). *Statistical package for the social sciences: SPSS^X.* New York: McGraw-Hill.

Wechsler, D. (1974). *Wechsler Intelligence Test for Children—Revised.* New York: Psychological Corporation.

Wepman, J. M. (1973). *Manual of administration, scoring, and interpretation: Auditory Discrimination Test Revised.* Los Angeles: Western Psychological Services.

Wood, M. M. (1986). *Developmental therapy.* Austin, TX: Pro-ed.

Zimet, S. G., & Farley, G. K. (1985). The self-concepts of children entering psychiatric day treatment. *Child Psychiatry and Human Development, 15,* 142–150.

Zimet, S. G., & Farley, G. K. (1986). Four perspectives on the competence and self-esteem of emotionally disturbed children beginning day treatment. *Journal of the American Academy of Child Psychiatry, 25,* 76–83.

Zimet, S. G., & Farley, G. K. (1987). How do emotionally disturbed children report on their competence and self-worth? *Journal of the American Academy of Child and Adolescent Psychiatry, 26,* 33–38.

Zimet, S. G., Farley, G. K., Silver, J., Hebert, F. B., Robb, E. D., Ekanger, C., & Smith, D. (1980). Behavior and personality changes in emotionally disturbed children enrolled in a psychoeducational day-treatment center. *Journal of the American Academy of Child Psychiatry, 19,* 240–252.

Zimet, S. G., Farley, G. K., & Dahlem, N. W. (1984). Behavior ratings of children in community schools and in day treatment. *International Journal of Partial Hospitalization, 2,* 199–208.

Zimet, S. G., Farley, G. K., & Dahlem, N. W. (1985). An abbreviated form of the WISC-R for use with emotionally disturbed children. *Psychology in the Schools, 22,* 19–22.

14

The Day Treatment Center as a Research Setting

A Review of Our Research

SARA GOODMAN ZIMET and GORDON K. FARLEY

INTRODUCTION

> The effect of health care services is becoming one of the most pressing issues for today's health policymakers. . . . There is mounting concern throughout the entire health care community that little is known about the relationship between many current clinical practices and . . . outcomes, about the impact of practitioners' diagnosis and treatment decisions on the health and well-being of their patients. (The Foundation for Health Services Research, 1989, p. 1)

What appears to be an imperative today—examining the quality of care provided in all modalities of mental health services—became a reality for us at the Day Care Center over 17 years ago, in 1973. That was the year that we established a comprehensive data base (see the Zimet, Farley, and Avitable chapter for a detailed description of this process), one of the few to be found in the United States. This move was prompted by both scholarly and clinical interests in the characteristics of children with serious emotional disorders. We were also curious about the process of change in various behavior and personality domains during and following treatment interventions.

The real beginnings of these interests can be traced back to 1967

SARA GOODMAN ZIMET and GORDON K. FARLEY • The Day Care Center, Department of Psychiatry, University of Colorado Health Sciences Center, Denver, Colorado 80262.

with the arrival of a new faculty member, a child psychiatrist, who joined the Day Care Center staff (Gordon K. Farley). He was successful in generating interest among two other faculty members—the center's director, Gaston E. Blom, a child psychiatrist and child psychoanalyst, and its chief social worker, Charles Ekanger—in carrying out a prospective study of the first 50 children who had been treated at the center. They were surprised to find that, although careful treatment progress notes were kept by teachers and clinical staff members, these notes were not standardized in form or content. In fact, no given piece of data except name, gender, date of birth, and the dates of entry to and discharge from the center was collected in the same way. Undaunted by this discovery, what had been planned as a prospective study became a retrospective one (Blom, Farley, & Ekanger, 1973).

The next step in carrying out program evaluation and research at our center was taken in 1973 when our child psychiatrist, Gordon K. Farley, became the center's director and Sara Goodman Zimet joined the faculty and center staff as director of research and program evaluation. The major goal of this partnership was to engage all the center's staff members in the design and implementation of a comprehensive data base. Within the year, the instruments were selected, the technicalities worked out, and the data collection, scoring, and recording begun. Five years later, complete data at four time points [entry (T1), discharge (T2), 6 months to 1 year following discharge (T3), and 1 year to 18 months after the first follow-up (T4)], on a group of approximately 52 children were available for analysis. The results of this first prospective follow-up study were presented in the *Journal of the American Academy of Child Psychiatry* (Zimet, Farley, Silver, Hebert, Robb, Ekanger, & Smith, 1980). This investigation set the stage for formulating hypotheses that would be tested a decade later when more subjects had been patients in our treatment program (Zimet, Farley, & Avitable, 1989).

In the interim years between 1978 and 1987, while our subject pool grew, our research focused on a variety of concerns. Some of the data were drawn from the data base, whereas other data were collected specifically for these projects. For example, we investigated the effect of five different methods of administering the Revised Wechsler Intelligence Scale for Children (WISC-R) (Jackson, Farley, Zimet, & Gottman, 1979); we developed an abbreviated form of the WISC-R (Zimet, Farley, & Dahlem, 1985); we examined the relationship between hearing acuity and auditory discrimination ability (Blager, 1978; Blager, Zimet, & Farley, 1983); we compared the school behavior ratings of teachers in public schools with those by our teachers on the same children (Zimet, Farley, & Dahlem, 1984); we explored self-concept ratings from a variety of approaches (Zimet & Farley, 1984, 1986, 1987); we studied the relationship between cortisol excretion and anxiety (Farley & Zimet, 1987a); we analyzed verbal samples to determine how well they predicted treatment outcome (Farley & Zimet, 1987b); and we investigated relationships with family and friends of a group of young adults who had been treated in our day hospital as children (Corkey & Zimet, 1987).

The methods and results of all of the studies inspired by our day treatment setting and outlined here are presented and discussed in the paragraphs that follow.

FOLLOW-UP STUDIES

Blom, Farley, and Ekanger, 1973

Our first follow-up study involved 50 children treated in our program for a mean length of time of 22 months. There were approximately three times as many boys as girls, and the majority were Caucasian (92%) with only 6% Afro-American, and 2% Hispanic. The GAP (Group for the Advancement of Psychiatry, 1966) diagnostic classifications included 2% autistic, 4% schizophreniform psychosis, 28% psychoneurosis, 50% personality disorder, 2% developmental deviation, and 14% borderline psychosis. The children were followed up at a mean length of time of 34 months after being discharged from day treatment. Forty-eight of the 50 children were located, and all of them agreed to participate in the study.

The measures we used and the sources of our information are outlined in Table 1.

We hypothesized that age at the time of entry to day treatment, parent involvement in treatment, and length of time in treatment would predict outcome at follow-up.

Table 1. Measures and Sources of Information

Measure	Sources of information		
	Chart review	Parents	Children
Symptom checklist	X	X	
Involvement in treatment	X		
Structured interview		X	X
Life events inventory		X	X
Satisfaction questionnaire		X	X

In brief, our findings were as follows:

1. Age was the only variable that demonstrated significant discriminating power between the good and the poor outcome groups. In effect, younger children were more likely to have better outcome ratings than older children. As a group, the children manifested problem behavior early in their school career, most by first grade. However, many of them were not referred to treatment until they were older.

2. Children diagnosed as borderline were described as well-adapted to their community classroom placements. Although these children still reported experiencing bizarre thoughts and fantasies, they nevertheless, were able to control them sufficiently so that their "imaginings" did not interfere with their day-to-day functioning.

3. Children with high normal and superior intelligence showed greater social improvement than academic achievement, despite the program's emphasis on academic work.

4. The majority of children tended to be indistinguishable from their peers. They had been described as "sore thumbs" at the time they entered our program. At follow-up, they now fitted in but were not outstanding in their school achievements.

5. There were no reports of delinquent behavior. One would expect a high rate of this behavior in such a population if they had been left untreated.

6. The children recalled their teachers by name but had difficulty remembering the names of their psychotherapists.

7. When asked about their satisfaction with the treatment they had received at our center, 98% of the families expressed positive attitudes. The patients' siblings, however, complained about the large amount of attention their brothers or sisters had received while they were in treatment with us.

Zimet, Farley, Silver, Hebert, Robb, Ekanger, and Smith, 1980

As indicated earlier, 5 years after we began collecting information systematically, we examined the records of those children on whom we had data covering the four check points: (a) entry to the center (T1); (b) discharge from the center (T2); (c) 6 months to 1 year after discharge (T3); and (d) 1 year to 18 months after the first follow-up (T4). There were 52 children who met these criteria. They were between the ages of 7 and 11 years old when they entered our center. There were three boys to every girl; 81% were Anglo, 17% were Afro-American, and 2% were Hispanic. The children were diagnosed using the GAP (Group for the Advancement of Psychiatry, 1966) classification system; 38% had person-

Table 2. Schedule of Information Collected on Each Child

Instrument	T1 Entry	T2 Termination	T3 First follow-up	T4 Second follow-up
School Behavior Checklist (Miller, 1977b)	X	X	X	X
Louisville Behavior Checklist (Miller, 1977a)	X	X	X	X
Wide Range Achievement Test (Jastak & Jastak, 1965)	X	X		X
Wechsler Intelligence Scale for Children–Revised (1974)	X	X		
Piers-Harris Children's Self-Concept Scale	X	X		

ality disorders; 32% had psychoneurotic disorders; 26% had developmental deviations; and 2% were diagnosed with reactive disorders and 2% with childhood psychoses. The purpose of this follow-up study was to examine the process and pattern of personality and behavior change over time during and following day psychiatric treatment.

An attempt was made to study several areas of the children's lives—their home and school behavior, academic achievement, intellectual performance, and self-esteem. The measures selected and the schedule for collecting the data are shown in Table 2. All assessment tools were chosen because they demonstrated the best validity and reliability available at the time and because age and/or sex norms had been established.

On average, data collection covered a period of approximately 2 years of treatment in the center, followed by another 2 years of posttreatment contacts, an average of approximately 4 years from the time day treatment was initiated. It was hypothesized that the children's behaviors and performance in each of the domains studied would improve over time.

A one-group pretest–posttest design was used. Differences between the scores obtained for each student on each of the measures during the four time periods were computed. The means of the differences for each measure were subjected to t tests, and a one-tailed test was used to determine the significance of the differences. We found that "the overall disability scores of home and school behaviors changed significantly in a positive direction between the time children began and terminated treatment (T1 vs. T2), and were maintained at the two follow-up points (T1 vs. T3 and T1 vs. T4)" (Zimet & Farley, 1985, p. 736).

Parents', teachers', and children's assessments over time appeared to parallel one another, suggesting a possible interactive relationship. Thus we assumed that the increase in positive ratings by parents and teachers would be accompanied by manifestations of greater acceptance toward the children and that the children, in turn, would report more positive perceptions about themselves. The data appeared to support this assumption.

> Children's self-reports of self-esteem . . . changed significantly in a positive direction by the end of day treatment (T1 vs. T2). Children reported themselves [at the beginning of day treatment to have adequate levels of self-esteem and at the end of day treatment] as having significantly more friends, looking more attractive, doing better in school work, feeling happier and less anxious, and as behaving better at school. (Zimet & Farley, 1985, p. 736)

The fact that the children, as a group, reported that they saw themselves in relatively positive terms at entry to day treatment was in contrast to how most clinicians believe children with serious emotional disorders view themselves. This finding intrigued us and led to the three studies reported later in this chapter (Zimet & Farley, 1984, 1986, and 1987).

The home behavior checklist (Miller, 1977a) ratings of each parent pair were compared. We found that mothers tended to see more deviant behaviors than fathers throughout the data-collection period. On the other hand, fathers reported significantly more attractive and desirable behaviors than did mothers.

As in the Blom, Farley, and Ekanger (1973) study described before, the children in the present study did not appear to make large gains in their academic skills, but neither did they stand still. The Academic Disability subscale of the School Behavior Checklist (Miller, 1977b) indicated that the children did not fall further behind in their academic performance, and the results of the Wide Range Achievement Test confirmed this finding.

> During the two-year enrollment at the Center, there was a significant gain of approximately two grades in reading . . . just under two grades in arithmetic . . . and approximately one and a half grades in spelling . . . This increase in performance begins to level off somewhat after termination, although gain scores between entry and final follow-up in arithmetic and reading continue to be significant. (Zimet et al., 1980, p. 245)

More recently, we have examined the academic profiles of our children over the four time periods in greater detail in an attempt to identify possible patterns of change and predictors of outcome (Zimet, Farley, & Avitable, 1989). The results are discussed later in this chapter under the heading, "Study of Achievement in Reading, Spelling, and Arithmetic."

We guessed that the improvement in academic performance might be linked to a change in the children's motivation to learn. Thus we examined the findings of the Low Need Achievement subscale of the School Behavior Checklist (Miller, 1977b). We did find a significant improvement between each time lapse: T1 to T2, T1 to T3, and T1 to T4.

A study by LaVietes and her associates (1965) found no significant change in IQ scores from the time day treatment began until it ended; however, a group of our children showed significant changes in IQ scale and subscale scores across those same time spans. We found "their highest T1 scores [to be] on the Performance rather than on the Verbal IQ Scale, [and] their largest increment at T2 . . . on the Performance IQ Scale" (Zimet & Farley, 1985, p. 736).

A finding of further interest is one that has been corroborated by other studies of children referred for psychological services (Glasser & Zimmerman, 1967)—that the Coding subtest produced the lowest scores. With our children, this was true at both T1 and T2. Arithmetic was another subtest in which the children performed poorly. Both Coding and Arithmetic along with Digit Span are the subtests identified by Kaufman (1975) as belonging to a Freedom from Distractibility factor. Low scores are believed to be typical of children with attention deficit disorders as defined by DSMIII-R criteria (American Psychiatric Association, 1987; Lufi & Cohen, 1985; Lufi, Cohen, & Parish-Plass, 1990). Low scores on these same subtests plus the Information subtest produce what is referred to as the ACID profile, which is said to be typical of learning-disabled children (Ackerman, Dykman, & Peters, 1976, 1977). Thus, as a consequence of these findings, we are eager to examine a larger group of our children for specific WISC-R performance patterns on Wechsler's (1974) and Kaufman's (1975) factors and also to see what changes might occur at the end of treatment with children exhibiting these patterns. Furthermore, we wondered if the intellectual performance of children placed in a day treatment setting would differ from those placed in an inpatient setting. These studies are presently underway.

An additional area of concern emerged as a result of these findings from the WISC-R (Wechsler, 1974). We wondered to what extent the procedures used to administer the test might effect performance (Jackson, Farley, Zimet, & Gottman, 1979), and if there was an abbreviated form of the WISC-R that might be used effectively to test this group of children (Zimet, Farley, & Dahlem, 1985; Zimet & Adler, 1990). The studies that emerged from these concerns are discussed later in this chapter under the heading, "Studies of Intelligence Testing." As a result of this prospective follow-up study, "Many questions . . . [were] raised regarding the length of time needed before behavioral changes are manifested, if and how long they are maintained, and which antecedent and

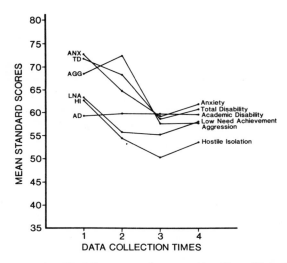

Figure 1. School Behavior Checklist mean scale scores. *Note.* From "Behavior and Personality Changes in Emotionally Disturbed Children in a Psychoeducational Day Treatment Center," by S. G. Zimet, G. K. Farley, J. Silver, F. B. Hebert, E. D. Robb, C. Ekanger, and D. Smith, 1980, *Journal of the American Academy of Child Psychiatry, 19,* p. 244. Copyright © 1980 by the American Academy of Child Psychiatry. Reprinted by permission.

intervening events are related to the time and durability of these changes" (Zimet & Farley, 1985, p. 737).

> Many researchers, in fact, have found that the outcome of psychotherapeutic interventions may become manifest well after the conclusion of treatment (Heinicke & Goldman, 1960; Lehrman, Sirluck, Black, & Glick, 1949; Levitt, 1957; Wright, Moelis, & Pollack, 1976). Furthermore, Lehrman [and his associates] . . . demonstrated that this *increment at follow-up phenomenon* is not due to temporal factors (e.g., normal developmental changes). Explanations for this pathway to a healthy adjustment may be found in the temporary regression associated with the termination process, and also to the time needed to transfer and integrate the skills and competencies learned in a treatment setting to a community setting.
>
> The *increment at follow-up phenomenon* in a day treatment setting is well illustrated in the more detailed school behavior data. . . . As shown in Figure 1, aggressive behavior ratings . . . increased from T1 to T2 and then decreased dramatically from T2 to T3; and anxious . . . withdrawn-hostile . . . behaviors and low motivation to learn . . . decreased from T2 to T3, showing no significant changes at T4. It also may be that the immediate effect of an intensive psychotherapeutic milieu is on the "deeper" structural aspects of personality functioning rather than in directly altering behavior. If this is true, then this personality reconstruction may pave the way for the later emergence of behavioral alterations and adaptations. (Zimet & Farley, 1985, p. 737)

Zimet, Farley, and Dahlem, 1984

Several methodological problems became salient during the planning and implementing of the prospective follow-up study described. The investigation now under review focuses on one such problem— observer bias. The potential impact of observer bias occurs when ratings are being made of the same children when the observational settings, the raters, and the raters' frame of reference are disparate. We wondered if behavior ratings done by public-school teachers would be similar to those done by our teachers because they each have very different reference groups with which to compare the children. Thus in order to determine the reliability of changes found in school behavior ratings at post-treatment follow-ups, the reliability of school behavior ratings by community-based teachers and day treatment teachers was studied using a test–retest paradigm.

Each of 49 children referred for day treatment to our center over an 8-year period was rated on the same standardized school behavior checklist (Miller, 1977b) by two teachers. One teacher was from their community classroom at the time of referral to day treatment, and one teacher was from our center 6 weeks later. There were 34 (69%) boys and 15 (31%) girls in the sample. Of these, 34 (69%) were white, 13 (27%) were Afro-American, and 2 (4%) were Hispanic. They ranged in age from 5.2 to 14.5 years old. Differences between teacher ratings and the effects of age and sex of the children on their ratings were examined using t tests of the mean difference scores. Relationships among subscale scores for each set of teachers and between teacher pairs were examined with Pearson product moment correlation coefficients.

No significant differences in mean scale scores were found between the two sets of teacher ratings. Correlation coefficients between scale scores of each teacher group ranged from moderately low (.20) to moderately high (.66). All but one comparison was significantly different from zero. Both teacher groups showed similar ratings when they were examined for age and gender of the children. The results suggest that school behavior ratings across teachers with very different frames of reference and from very different classroom settings are likely to provide an acceptable index of behavior change at posttreatment follow-up.

Corkey and Zimet, 1987

In the process of pursuing her doctoral studies at Smith College School of Social Work, Caroline Corkey, one of the social work faculty members on our center staff, decided to examine the relationships with family and friends of our expatients who were now young adults between the ages of 18 and 25 years old. Sara Goodman Zimet, as adjunct professor at Smith College, was her dissertation advisor. Because this study is presented in its entirety in the next chapter, only a brief review is offered below.

Fifty-one of the center's past patients met the age criteria. Of these, 48.2% were available and willing to participate in the study. When the obtained and lost subjects were compared, no significant differences between them were found regarding entry age to day treatment, length of time in treatment, and distribution by gender and by race. On the other hand, the obtained sample were older when they left day treatment, had a shorter time lapse between discharge and follow-up, and included more subjects who were severely disturbed as children than did the lost sample. Furthermore, all three subjects with severe organicity were in the obtained sample. Because of these conditions, we expected our findings to be biased against a positive outcome. Nevertheless, it was hypothesized that the majority of young adults studied would have achieved developmentally appropriate interpersonal relationships with parents, significant others, and friends. Because sex roles are differentiated along the lines of interpersonal relationships, we expected that the female young adults would demonstrate a more mature stage of development than their male counterparts. Furthermore, we expected to find the severity of the emotional disorder and age at the time of entry to day treatment to be significantly related to interpersonal relationships in young adulthood.

Data were collected during individual 2-hour semistructured interviews. Transcripts of the interviews were scored using three rating scales: (a) one tapping relationships with parents (Blatt, Chevron, Quinlan, & Wein, 1981); (b) another characterizing relationships with friends and developed by Corkey; and (c) the third describing the support seen as available from family, significant others, and friends (Zimet, Dahlem, Zimet, & Farley, 1988). The data were also examined by severity of the emotional disturbance, extent of organicity, and age at entry.

Comparisons were made with the standardization population on the parent relationship measure (Blatt, Chevron, Quinlan, & Wein, 1981) using t tests. Relationships between measures and variables were examined using a one-way analysis of variance, chi-square tests, and Pearson product moment correlation coefficients.

Despite the potential bias against a positive outcome, the majority of young adults were at developmentally appropriate levels in their interpersonal relationships with parents, friends, and significant others. In addition, most of them felt that they had recourse to a substantial level of support from the significant people in their lives. The expectation that females would be at a more mature level than males was not supported.

We were surprised to find that the young adults in this study sample and the young adults who were among the standardization sample for the measure devised by Blatt and his colleagues (1981) were more similar than different in their relationships with their parents.

> As predicted, an early age at entry to day treatment appeared to be significantly related to more mature perceptions of relationships with parents in young adulthood. These findings lend support to results from . . . [the first follow-up study reviewed here carried out by Blom, Farley, and Ekanger (1973)] . . . Similarly, Prentice-Dunn and his colleagues (1981) found that children who showed the most positive behavioral changes were youngest when day psychiatric treatment was begun. (Corkey & Zimet, 1987, p. 111)

PREDICTIVE STUDIES

Farley and Zimet, 1987a

We wondered to what extent urinary-free cortisol excretion (UFCE) assessed from urine samples collected on days designated as stressful would reflect certain psychological states measured at the time the children entered our treatment program. Our subjects were 15 children with a mean age of 9.4 years; four were girls and 11 were boys. The two events designated as stressors were the first day of the study and Halloween day. Seven urine samples were obtained from each child over a period of 6 consecutive weeks. One specimen was collected the first, third, fourth, fifth, and sixth weeks, and two were collected the second week, the week Halloween was celebrated. Each specimen represented the total volume of urine excreted between 9 A.M. and 11 A.M. Urinary-free cortisol was determined by a radioimmunoassay method. Levels of cortisol excretion were expressed in three ways: (a) micrograms cortisol per minute, (b) micrograms cortisol per minute per square meter of body surface, and (c) micrograms cortisol per milligrams creatinine.

Anxiety was measured in three ways: (a) by teachers' ratings of anxiety on the School Behavior Checklist (Miller, 1977b); (b) children's self-ratings on the General Anxiety Scale for Children (Sarason, Davidson, Lighthall, Waite, & Ruebush, 1960); and (c) a Halloween Fear Scale developed by Zimet and Farley. Intelligence was measured by the WISC-R FSIQ (Wechsler, 1974) and by the cognitive scale of the Perceived Competence Scale for Children (Harter, 1978). The Total Disability score of Miller's (1977b) School Behavior Checklist was our measure of severity of the children's psychopathology. Finally, significant life events occurring at the children's home during the 6 weeks of the data collection were recorded by the parent and/or family therapists.

No relationship was found between UFCE levels and any of the measures of psychological status at T1. In addition, there was no significant increase in UFCE levels on the designated stress days or from week-to-week for most children. A rise in UFCE occurred with the advent of a significant life event for some children but not for others. Surprisingly, significantly lower levels of cortisol were excreted by children who perceived themselves as being low in general anxiety and more competent in their academic work. When lean body weight was taken into account, girls showed significantly higher UFCE levels than boys, and older children had higher UFCE levels than younger children. Furthermore, there was no association demonstrated between teachers' ratings and children's ratings of anxiety or between WISC-R (Wechsler, 1974) IQ scores and perceived cognitive competence. In effect, our findings appear to indicate that UFCE was not a reliable indicator of the psychological status of a group of children entering day psychiatric treatment.

Farley and Zimet, 1987b

We attempted to predict outcome of day treatment at discharge (T2) and at a 18-to-24-month follow-up (T4) from a content analysis of 62 children's 5-minute verbal samples obtained at the time they entered our center (T1). The technique of obtaining and scoring verbal samples for a broad variety of psychological states was developed by Gottschalk and his associates (Gottschalk, 1974, 1976, 1982; Gottschalk, Uliana, & Hoigaard, 1979). As predictors, we used verbal sample scales of Hope, Human Relations, and Cognitive Impairment. As outcome measures, we used changes on the Severity Level, Aggression, Inhibition, Neurotic, Rare Deviance, and Academic Disability scales of the Miller (1977a) Home Behavior Checklist. For more discrete analyses, we divided the children into two groups, those classified as organically impaired and those who were not organically impaired. The designations were made using five neurobehavioral signs selected by Gordon K. Farley. Those children who were rated as having three or more of these signs at T1 were classified as organically impaired.

We discovered that verbal sample analysis on the three scales provided only modestly accurate predictors of improvement. Of the three scales, Cognitive Impairment was the best predictor of outcome, particularly with children who were not grossly organically impaired. It is of interest to note that organicity also contributed to a less mature relationship with friends and family in young adulthood in the Corkey and

Zimet (1987) follow-up study and in a poorer outcome in academic achievement in the Zimet, Farley, and Avitable (1989) investigation.

STUDIES OF COMPETENCE AND SELF-ESTEEM

Zimet and Farley, 1984, 1986, 1987

Most mental health theorists and practitioners have assumed that children with serious emotional disorders are likely to perceive themselves negatively and therefore as inadequate in most areas of their lives (Mead, 1934; Rogers, 1951; Sullivan, 1953). Our own clinical experience with children in day treatment supported this assumption. The children frequently said that they hated themselves and referred to themselves as stupid, unloved by their families, and as having no friends. Furthermore, these feelings tended to be validated by their life experiences. They were likely to have failed repeatedly in school subjects, and they were frequently rejected by parents, siblings, teachers, and/or peers. Thus when we found that their self-reports indicated that they felt relatively good about themselves (see review of the Zimet *et al.,* 1980 follow-up study), we decided to examine the literature. The research that was available indicated that, whereas the self-concepts of clinic-referred children differed significantly from those of normal children, their scores were still within the normal range and therefore not as clinically significant as had been assumed. We did notice, however, that the scores of the children with emotional disorders had higher variances than those of normal children, indicating that their scores covered a wider range, more at the lower and upper ends of the scale.

The First Study. We decided to examine this issue with 68 children beginning day treatment (Zimet & Farley, 1984) by comparing them with groups of normal and clinic-referred children studied by others (Bloom, Shea, & Eun, 1979; Piers, 1972) using the same instrument, the Piers-Harris Self-Concept Scale for Children (Piers, 1969). We also examined the possible influence on self-concept ratings of gender, SES (Hollingshead & Redlich, 1958) and severity of the emotional disorder as measured by the Total Disability Scale of Miller's (1977b) School Behavior Checklist. Our prediction that children in day treatment would have significantly lower self-concepts scores than normal and clinic-referred children was not met. In fact, a trend in the opposite direction emerged. We found that only 25% of the children perceived themselves in strongly disparaging terms and we called these children "disparagers." The remaining 75% were split between those who saw themselves as normal children do, "positivists," and those whose self-concepts were highly inflated, "extollers." The mean self-concept scores of day treatment children did not differ significantly from those of normal children. However, there was a trend toward a significant difference between day treatment and clinic-referred children. In fact, our children had the higher scores.

The results from a within-group analysis of our children's scores regarding severity of emotional disorder were in contrast to the between-group analysis. The greater the severity scores, the lower the self-concepts scores. SES was also found to be associated with self-perceptions: The lower the SES, the lower the self-concept scores. On the other hand, IQ, sex, and race did not appear to influence self-concept ratings.

We were very surprised to learn that the findings from the prospective follow-up study were confirmed and that our clinical observations of the children's self-perceptions did not match their own reports. It may have been that we were being overly influenced by the 25% who were disparagers. We also wondered if we would get a wider range of scores if the children were rated by the significant adults in their lives on the same scale used by the children. It also occurred to us that our observations may have been valid but that most of the children were actively engaged in denying the realities of their lives as a way of trying to cope with them. Finally, we were concerned about the nature of the PHS (Piers, 1969), the measure we had been using. Its format appeared to enhance the tendency of young children to describe themselves in more positive terms. In order to answer some of these questions, we designed the following two studies: (a) one that compared the self-reports of children in day treatment on two different self-concept measures, the PHS and the Perceived Competence Scale for Children (PCSC; Harter, 1978); and (b) one that examined four views of the child's competence and self-worth: the child's, the primary caretaker's, the teacher's, and the child's psychotherapist, using the PCSC only.

The Second Study. The primary purpose of this investigation (Zimet & Farley, 1987) was to compare the children's ratings of self-esteem on two instruments, one whose format was believed to draw socially desirable responses [the PHS (Piers, 1969)], and one whose format was especially designed to reduce this tendency of young children to describe themselves in more socially acceptable terms [the PCSC (Harter, 1978)]. We were also interested in comparing our subjects with Harter's California/Connecticut standardization sample and to determine, with this new instrument, whether children in day psychiatric treatment differentiated among the four domains of their lives tapped by the PCSC (academic competence, popularity with peers, athletic ability, and general self-

Table 3. Characteristics of Children in Day Treatment Taking the Piers-Harris Scale (PHS)[a] and the Perceived Competence Scale for Children (PCSC)[b]

Characteristics	PHS	PCSC
Age (years)		
M	9.60	10.38
SD	1.78	2.21
Sex (%)		
Girls	27.9	32.4
Boys	72.1	67.6
Severity		
M	73.76	71.76
SD	13.19	15.75
SES		
M	3.37	3.18
SD	1.51	1.53
IQ: Full scale		
M	90.13	91.38
SD	13.87	17.31

[a]$N = 68$.
[b]$N = 34$.
Note. From "How Do Emotionally Disturbed Children Report Their Competencies and Self-Worth?", by S. G. Zimet and G. K. Farley, 1987, *Journal of the American Academy of Child and Adolescent Psychiatry*, 26, p. 34. Copyright 1987 by the American Academy of Child and Adolescent Psychiatry. Reprinted by permission.

worth), as most normal children do in this age range. Examining this kind of issue was not possible with the PHS because only a total self-concept score could be obtained.

Two groups of children entering our day treatment center at two different time periods (1973–1977 and 1978–1983) were the subjects of this second study (Zimet & Farley, 1987). Group 1 ($N = 68$) completed the PHS (Piers, 1969) and Group 2 ($N = 34$), the PCSC (Harter, 1978). The two groups did not differ significantly from each other in age, gender, severity, SES, or intelligence (see Table 3 for these data). The same measures of these variables used in the first study were used in this study, although the Full Scale IQ score was used in place of either the Verbal or Performance IQ scores.

Surprisingly, both self-concept measures drew primarily positive answers from the children. In effect, the findings from this study support the general findings from ... [our first] study that most of the ... children ... see themselves in primarily positive terms. The majority of girls and boys report themselves to be very competent in their school work, very popular with their peers, very adept at sports, and they value themselves highly. [Their scores indicate that they see themselves as] ... athletically superior to their normal counterparts. In addition, most ... [of these children], as compared to normal children, seem to view themselves more

globally than multidimensionally, suggesting that they are responding like children
who are functioning at an earlier stage of development (Silon, 1980; Harter, 1982).
   While a majority of . . . children fell in the combined group of positivists and
extollers, one quarter met the criterion for the disparager group. Both patterns of
self-denigration and self-aggrandizement are believed by the authors to be maneu-
vers to protect the self from the ridicule of others as well as to obviate one's own
disappointment at failing to achieve the goals set by the self and/or by significant
others. (Zimet & Farley, 1987, p. 36)

   None of the other variables studied (sex, severity of the disorder,
intelligence, or SES), was related to self-concept ratings.

   The questions that still remained to be answered were (a) how
would adults who knew the children well rate them on the four scales of
the PCSC (Harter, 1978), and (b) how would their ratings compare to
those of the children's?

   The Third Study. At the same time that the 34 children described in
the second study were given the PCSC (Harter, 1978), we asked each of
the children's primary caretaker, psychotherapist, and teacher to rate
the child the way he or she perceived the child's competencies and self-
worth, *not* the way each thought the child would rate him- or herself.

   It will be recalled that the main purpose of this third study (Zimet &
Farley, 1986) was to determine what the areas of agreement and disagreement were among the four rater groups, not simply to identify
which group reported most accurately. Based on our earlier studies, we
made several predictions. First, we predicted that children's scores
would be the highest of all rater groups. Their tendency to answer in a
socially desirable direction would prevail either because the self-reveal-
ing nature of the questions would provoke enough anxiety to mobilize
their defenses or because unconditional acceptance in the treatment
center might evoke optimism and hope that the pattern of past rejec-
tions and failures had been broken. Second, we predicted that differences among adults would be small because there was so much communication among them within the center. Third, on the basis of the
differences in role functions of each adult group with the children, we
predicted that the ranking of adult raters' scores would be highest for
caretakers, lowest for teachers, and psychotherapists' scores would fall
between parents' and teachers' scores.

   Because we found SES and severity of disorder to be related to self-
concept scores in our first study, we continued to include these two
variables for investigation particularly as they related to adult raters'
scores, again using the same measures as in the first study. We were also
curious to see if the ratings of the children's cognitive competence were
at all related to the children's Verbal and/or Performance IQ scores.

   All of our predictions were supported. We found a consistent rank-

Table 4. Means, Standard Deviations, and Rank Order of Scale Scores of Four Rater Groups

Scale	Children	Caretakers	Psychotherapists	Teachers
Physical				
M	3.24	2.75	2.81	2.52
SD	0.83	0.87	0.77	0.89
Rank				
Down	1	2	1	2
Across	1	3	2	4
Social				
M	3.12	2.51	2.19	2.09
SD	0.83	0.92	0.81	0.93
Rank				
Down	2	3	3	3
Across	1	2	3	4
Cognitive				
M	3.03	2.78	2.62	2.55
SD	0.75	0.79	0.86	0.85
Rank				
Down	3	1	2	1
Across	1	2	3	4
General				
M	2.84	2.06	2.05	2.04
SD	0.87	0.86	0.65	0.75
Rank				
Down	4	4	4	4
Across	1	2	3	4

Note. From "Four Perspectives on the Competence and Self-Esteem of Emotionally Disturbed Children Beginning Day Treatment," by S. G. Zimet and G. K. Farley, 1986, *Journal of the American Academy of Child Psychiatry, 25,* p. 79. Copyright 1986 by the American Academy of Child Psychiatry. Reprinted by permission.

ing pattern of raters across the four scales. Children rated themselves as most competent, followed by parents, next therapists, and then teachers. Adult raters' scores were also ranked in the predicted sequence. The means, standard deviations, and rank order of scale scores within and across rater groups may be seen in Table 4.

All of the children's scores were well above the theoretical mean of the Perceived Competence Scale (Harter, 1978) and higher than those of the normative sample. In effect, children, as a group, tended to overrate their own competencies when compared to adult raters who are presumably somewhat more objective. Furthermore, adult raters did not differ from each other appreciably, but they did differ from the way children rated themselves. From an analysis of variance, we found significant differences among raters on all scales. A *post hoc* test indicated that significant differences were found between children and teachers and children and their primary caretakers; there was also a trend toward a significant difference between children and their therapists. These findings appear to lend credence to the contribution of role theory to our prediction. We found no correspondence between children's ratings of their cognitive ability and Verbal IQ Scale scores. The opposite was true with the adult raters, where the correlations ranged from moderate and significant (caretakers) to strong and significant (psychotherapists and teachers).

Unlike Harter (1978), we did not find gender differences on children's own ratings of their athletic abilities. A sex difference in boys and girls ratings was found on the social scale, however. Boys saw themselves as being more popular than girls saw themselves. In contrast, caretakers of girls gave them higher ratings on the social scale then did caretakers of boys. Neither teachers nor therapists distinguished between boys and girls in any of their ratings.

The severity of the children's emotional disorders appeared to influence teachers and caretakers' ratings in the expected direction. The higher the severity level score, the lower the competence and self-worth scores. This was not the case for children or for their psychotherapists.

Unlike our first study, neither SES nor age were significantly related to competence and self-worth ratings by either the children or the adult rater groups.

In order to determine the extent to which the aforementioned variables that were found to be significantly different from zero may have contributed to explaining the variance in the PCSC scale scores, a stepwise multiple regression analysis was carried out. For children's ratings, none of the variables contributed in any important way to their views of themselves. In contrast, however, it appears that the adult groups were using information about the children on which a sizable proportion of the ratings were based. Verbal intelligence, gender, and severity of the disorder influenced caretakers; verbal intelligence and severity effected psychotherapists; and performance and verbal intellectual abilities, severity level, and gender contributed to teachers' ratings. "It has been suggested that the ability of emotionally disturbed children to assess themselves accurately is impaired by their emotional disorder (Wolman, 1972). This explanation fits in well with [our] observations . . . that, in general, these children do have difficulty in realistically assessing their competencies" (Zimet & Farley, 1986, pp. 82–83).

It would be of interest to determine if children are better judges of their abilities and self-worth by the time they are discharged from our treatment center. We found in our first prospective follow-up study that our children's PHS (Piers, 1969) scores increased significantly over the period from entry to termination (T1–T2). However, because the PHS currently has standardized scale scores in addition to the total scale score (Piers, 1984), we have decided to reexamine our data using an additional 20 subjects. We will also analyze the scores of our three self-concept groups at entry to day treatment, the disparagers, positivists, and extollers, to try to determine with greater specificity which group of children are likely to show the most improvement in self-assessment.

STUDY OF ACHIEVEMENT IN READING, SPELLING, AND ARITHMETIC

Zimet, Farley, and Avitable, 1989

There is much that we do not know regarding children's academic performance over time. For example, we do not know what happens to emotionally disturbed children who are having difficulties in academic work where no intervention versus intensive teaching and/or tutoring is provided. The assumption is that, without an intensive intervention, they will continue on a downward spiral. We do not know what kind of progress to expect of children with specified base rates. In effect, we are just at the forefront of investigating patterns of growth and change in academic functioning among normal and emotionally disturbed children (Alexander & Entwisle, 1988; Feshbach & Feshbach, 1987).

As discussed earlier, we had found from our prospective follow-up study (Zimet *et al.,* 1980) that our children, as a group, did progress in reading and arithmetic during the time they were in treatment and at the follow-up testing approximately 2 years later. In the study now described, we set out to further explore the academic performance of a larger group of children who had complete Wide Range Achievement Test (WRAT) (Jastak & Jastak, 1978) scores in reading, spelling, and arithmetic over three testing times: entry to day treatment (T1), discharge from day treatment (T2), and follow-up approximately 18 months to 2 years after discharge (T4). (We did not collect the WRAT data at T3. From a total of 119 children enrolled at our center from 1973 to 1983, 87 met this criteria for reading and arithmetic and 78 for spelling. We were primarily concerned with two issues: (a) how do children, defined by their performance level at entry to day treatment, progress in each of the subject areas over the treatment period and at a follow-up time; and (b) what factors appear to contribute to this pathway. The factors studied included intelligence (WISC-R) (Wechsler, 1974), socioeconomic status (SES) (Hollingshead & Redlich, 1958), organic impairment (our own five categories), adjustment level [Global Assessment of Functioning Scale (GAF) from the DSM III-R (American Psychiatric Association, 1987)], school behavior [School Behavior Checklist (Miller, 1977b)], family living situation (FLS) (our own four categories), and length of time in treatment (number of days attended from entry to termination).

Each child was placed in one of the following three performance groups for each of the three academic subjects, based on their WRAT (Jastak & Jastak, 1978) score: (a) Normal and Above (NA), scores ≥ 85; (b) Moderately Impaired (MI), scores 70 to 84; and (c) Severely Impaired (SI), scores ≤ 69. We wondered if each child's performance across the three academic subjects was consistent enough to combine the three into one academic achievement factor. As a result of several analyses, we concluded that we should examine achievement in each of the three subject areas separately.

The following three performance outcome groups for each academic subject were also established, based on their WRAT (Jastak & Jastak, 1978) scores at T2 and T4: (a) Got Better, gained 15 points over the T1 score; (b) Progressed Evenly, remained within 15 points of the T1 score; and (c) Got Worse, lost 15 points from the T1 score.

Change of achievement test scores over the two time periods was examined using a change score (T2 mean minus T1 mean; T4 mean minus T1 mean). A multivariate repeated measures design was used to test for significant main and interaction effects. If significant effects were found, a one-way analysis of variance (ANOVA) was employed, followed by Fischer's Least Significant Difference multiple comparison procedure. Relationships between and among variables were examined using a chi-square test for categorical variables and one- and two-way ANOVAs, paired t tests, and Pearson product moment correlation coefficients for continuous variables. A z statistic was used to examine differences between correlations of independent samples. Additional *post hoc* analyses were carried out as needed. Finally, a stepwise multiple regression analysis was utilized to predict which of a selected group of variables at entry to day treatment contributed to reading, spelling, and arithmetic achievement test scores at termination and follow-up of day treatment.

The principal results of our investigation across academic subjects are summarized next:

1. Children in the NA groups were brighter, better functioning, less organically impaired, and were in treatment for a shorter period of time than children in the MI and SI academic performance groups.

Most of the children tended to be in either the NA or MI groups; very few were in the SI group.

2. The majority of children progressed evenly across time; very small proportions either deteriorated or improved in their academic performance. Of those who did get better, more came from the SI groups proportionately than from either the NA or MI groups, providing support for the concept of regression toward the mean for extreme groups. Alternatively, this suggests that some children in the SI group responded well to intensive treatment. Furthermore, SI change scores tended to be larger than those from the other academic performance groups. Achievement in the three subject areas appears to be highly stable over a 2-year period; arithmetic test scores less so than either reading or spelling, however. These findings are similar to those reported by Feshbach and Feshbach (1987) for reading and spelling with normal children.

3. The correlation coefficients between achievement test scores and FSIQ, GAF scores, organic impairment scores, and length of time in treatment tended to be moderate to strong and significantly different from zero. The higher the achievement test score, the higher the child's intelligence, the better his or her level of functioning, the less likelihood there was of organicity, and the shorter was his or her length of treatment time in our center. A comparison between the correlation coefficients obtained between the FSIQ and achievement test scores of our children and of the WRAT standardization sample resulted in significant differences with reading and spelling but with weaker associations obtained by our children across the three academic areas.

4. In keeping with the concept of persistence forecasting, the single best predictor of reading and spelling performance at termination from treatment and at follow-up was academic performance at entry to treatment. For arithmetic, it was both academic performance and intelligence as measured at the time the child entered our center.

STUDIES OF INTELLIGENCE TESTING

Jackson, Farley, Zimet, and Gottman, 1979

From our experience in testing children with serious emotional disorders, there were many occasions when it was necessary to modify the standard administrative procedures in order to get what we considered to be a valid measure of the child's intellectual abilities. These modifications in procedures might focus on helping the child to be more attentive to the task and encouraging the child to continue to work and do his or her best in answering the questions using positive verbal reinforcements. We did not know, however, if our efforts actually made a difference in the children's test performance. In order to check this out systematically, we decided to examine the effects of five test administration conditions on the WISC-R (Wechsler, 1974) performance of low- and high-impulsive children most of whom were in day psychiatric treatment. In addition to the standard administration described in the test manual, our procedures included two that provided monetary reward for both attention to the task at hand and for success in completing the task, one providing feedback on success and failure and one that coached the children to use a self-vocalization procedure to orient their attention.

Children were identified as being low or high in impulsivity using the Porteus Maze Test (Porteus, 1942) and randomly assigned to each of the five administrative conditions. The conditions were compared using an overall analysis of variance and several 2 × 5 analyses of variance procedures.

A strong relationship was demonstrated between WISC-R (Wechsler, 1974) scores and administrative procedures. *Post hoc* analyses indicated that conditions that provide knowledge of success and those in which payment is given for desired behaviors were powerful motivators for improving the test performance of emotionally disturbed boys and high-impulsive children. Conversely, emotionally disturbed girls and low-impulsive children performed best when given information on the success of their performance.

Zimet, Farley, and Dahlem, 1985

We felt that there were several good reasons to identify a reliable and valid short form of the WISC-R (Wechsler, 1974) for use with children who had serious emotional disorders, such as those who were in our day treatment program. Two of the primary reasons are the difficulty these children have in keeping with a task and the need we have for updating assessments during the treatment period. Keeping in mind the limitations of such an instrument and the clinical responsibilities associated with evaluation procedures, we began our search for such an instrument. A review of the literature led us to testing the efficacy of two multiple regression derived, selected-subtest short forms using 101 full WISC-R test protocols of children enrolled in our center since 1973. (This review has recently been updated and published by Zimet & Adler, 1990.)

No significant differences were found between the mean IQ scale score of either of the short forms and the Full Scale IQ. Correlation coefficients were highly significant, ranging from .958 to .997. Furthermore, only one child shifted IQ classifications when using the short forms. Thus both short-form models provided time-saving estimates of the general intellectual performance of these children.

STUDIES OF HEARING AND AUDITORY DISCRIMINATION

Blager, 1978 and Blager, Zimet, and Farley, 1983

Children in our center who demonstrated unusual problems with attention and who performed poorly on the Wepman (1973) Auditory Discrimination Test were referred to Florence Blager, an audiologist on the faculty of the University of Colorado Health Sciences Center, for a diagnostic evaluation. During her many years of experience testing our children and others referred to her who had serious emotional disorders, she observed that some of them had an unusual pattern of performance on an auditory discrimination test. They performed better in noise than in quiet. In consulting the literature, she found no studies examining this issue with children. The norms presented in the Goldman–Fristoe–Woodcock Test of Auditory Discrimination (GFW) (Goldman, Fristoe, & Woodcock, 1970), however, showed two populations better in noise than in quiet: the hard of hearing and the culturally disadvantaged. Neither of these groups was described as also having serious emotional disorders. Attempts to investigate these observations resulted in the two studies described next.

The First Study. Eighteen children between 6 and 13 years old, who were enrolled in our center, were the subjects for this exploratory study. The following questions were asked: (a) would the center children respond to the GFW the same as normal children do; and (b) would the center children respond better in the noise condition than in the quiet condition. Each child was individually administered the GFW, using both the quiet and noise conditions by Florence Blager in a carefully controlled testing environment. Percentile rank scores of center children were compared to those of the GFW normative sample by applying the Wilcoxon Matched-Pairs Signed-Ranks test followed by a one-tailed test of significance.

Our center children showed a median score and interquartile range in both the quiet and noise conditions that was quite different from the normative sample's. Thus the center's children did not respond to the GFW in the same way as normal children respond. Our center children performed at a level closer to the norms for the poor discriminators as described in the test manual (Goldman, Fristoe, & Woodcock, 1970).

When comparing their performances in the quiet versus the noise conditions, however, the center children, as a group, did not respond differently from the children in the standardization sample. From an examination of the test protocols, 6 of the 18 children did perform better in noise than in quiet, an occurrence that was more frequent than would be expected by chance alone. Blager speculated that the background noise may have either acted to mask the children's "internal noise" or that listening in the noise condition required maximal attention and resulted in improved performance in those children able to exert that attention. However, because this study was the only one suggesting that there may be a subgroup of children with serious emotional problems whose auditory discrimination abilities are less impaired by noise, Blager decided that a replication of this study should be attempted, one that would include additional information on the subjects and would examine the relationship of other variables to the children's performance on the GFW. At this point, Sara Goodman Zimet and Gordon K. Farley joined with Florence Blager in carrying out the second study.

The Second Study. At the time of this study, there were 17 children enrolled at the center who were between the ages of 8 and 12 years old. Both vision and hearing tests were individually administered, and the children were found to be in the normal range on both tests. As in the previous study, the GFW was individually administered under controlled testing conditions. The center children's GFW (Goldman, Fristoe, & Woodcock, 1970) percentile scores were compared to those in the GFW manual for normal discriminators, poor discriminators, hard of hearing, and culturally disadvantaged children. The tests were scored for both quiet and noise conditions. In addition to the analyses carried out in the first study, other approaches were used as well. For example, the children were separated into two groups: (a) those who had relatively higher percentile rank scores in the quiet condition ($N = 10$); and (b) those who had relatively higher percentile rank scores in the noise condition ($N = 7$); then these groups were compared as to their performance in the two conditions. The other analyses used are discussed in the context of the findings.

As in the first study and despite normal hearing acuity, this group of children's performance was similar to that of the "poor discriminators" described in the GFW manual (Goldman, Fristoe, & Woodcock, 1970). They had lower than average percentile rank scores in both quiet and noise conditions. However, when the Wilcoxon Matched-Pairs Sign test was applied, the earlier findings were not replicated. The children who did relatively better in the noise condition did not perform significantly better in the noise condition than children who did relatively better in the quiet condition. The data were reanalyzed using a *t* test of mean difference scores, and the lack of support for the findings of the first study was confirmed. Furthermore, we found that the scores of the noise and quiet conditions subtests were moderately correlated in these data. Whereas in the first study, the correlations were poor, "the inability to replicate the [original] findings suggested that there might have been important differences in Ss. . . . Comparisons of the . . . demographic and personality characteristics were investigated using a chi square test and *t* tests . . . with [a] two-tailed test of significance" (Blager, Zimet, & Farley, 1983, p. 80).

No differences were found between the two subject groups on GFW scores by sex, age, intelligence, or severity of emotional disorder. Thus the inability to replicate the findings of the first study cannot be explained by differences in these characteristics.

Several questions were raised regarding the reliability and validity of the GFW (Goldman, Fristoe, & Woodcock, 1970) as a result of the two studies. For example, there was some indication from an examination of the mean scores shown in the GFW manual for their standardization population that having higher percentile rank scores in the noise versus the quiet condition may not be an unusual occurrence. In addition, doubts were raised regarding the process of transforming raw scores to percentile rank scores. The addition or deletion of 1 point can shift the percentile rank scores significantly. Finally, we were concerned about the stability of GFW test scores with children who have serious emotional disorders. There was no information in the manual regarding this issue.

If we were to take the GFW (Goldman, Fristoe, & Woodcock, 1970) test results at face value, we would have to say that our daily observations of this sample of seriously emotionally disordered children is congruent with the test results. Despite normal hearing ability, they are not able to attend as well as normal children to tasks requiring judgment based on verbal cues.

SUMMARY AND CONCLUSIONS

There are several variables at the time of entry to day treatment (T1) that have been identified in more than one of our studies as being related to a favorable outcome at the time children leave day treatment (T2) and/or at follow-up times (T3 and/or T4). One of these is the age at which our children start day treatment. The younger they are, the better the outcome. This speaks to the issue of early identification, in preschool and kindergarten, of children who require intensive therapeutic treatment interventions. In addition, it raises the issue of what kinds of interventions might be more effective in the habilitation and rehabilitation of older school-age children. Two other variables identified by us are the severity of the child's emotional disorder and the extent of the child's organicity. Children with less severe emotional disorders and lower levels of organicity appear to be in treatment over a shorter period of time and make greater gains overall than children with higher levels of severity of psychopathology and organicity. As with the older children, these children may require different kinds of intense therapeutic interventions than the ones we are currently providing, such as more structured behavior modification programs across the social, affective, and educational areas, as well as the introduction of physical and occupational therapy as an integral part of our treatment program.

In general terms, we found that significant positive gains were made by our children over time in several areas of their lives. Teachers rated children as improving significantly in their behavior at school, and we found that we could rely on teachers ratings as an index of outcome. Most of the children no longer stood out as sore thumbs but appeared, instead, to be indistinguishable from the other children in their community school classrooms. Although we did find that children did not make large gains in their academic skills, neither did they fall further behind nor did they stand still. The majority of children progressed evenly throughout the period of treatment and two follow-ups. At all assessment times, the children's highest scores were in reading, next spelling, and last arithmetic.

Parents, both fathers and mothers, also reported a significant improvement in behaviors at home. Fathers tended to rate their children more positively than mothers. Intellectual ability also appeared to improve significantly, particularly in the performance domain.

Regardless of the test used to measure self-concept, the children tended to answer questions about themselves in primarily positive terms at the beginning and at the end of treatment. At discharge from treatment, nevertheless, they reported having more friends, feeling less anxious, looking more attractive, doing better in their school behavior and in their schoolwork, and feeling happier than when they entered our Center. Furthermore, at the beginning of treatment, children tended to perceive their abilities and general self-worth quite differently than did the significant adults in their lives. Children's self-assessments were highest, followed by their primary caretakers', psychotherapists', and teachers' assessments. Although most children tend to rate themselves positively, emotionally disturbed children appear to have more difficulty than normal children in evaluating their strengths and weaknesses. This problem suggests some special effort be placed in the treatment program to help these children set more realistic goals for themselves.

In this review of the research carried out at our center, the reader can see how one study led to another and together form some important pieces of a puzzle. We have recognized the need to check out our "clinical hunches" and to withhold judgment regarding these hunches until we have firmer ground to stand on. Our work has reminded us frequently, how difficult it is to get a clear-cut, straightforward answer to what we believed to be relatively simple clinical questions. Although there are considerable obstacles to this work, including staff resistance or apathy (see a discussion of the human factor in the data base chapter), limited funding availability (see the chapter on funding a day treatment program), and equivocal findings, we believe that we have demonstrated that it is still possible to produce important work. Useful data have been generated. Our studies have been used to support the efficacy of the day treatment modality with a number of insurers, state agencies, legislative bodies, and department and university administrators.

We have also discovered through our research and program evaluation efforts what areas of our program need to be modified or replaced to increase the effectiveness of our interventions. Although the methodological problems facing clinical researchers are formidable at times, there are very good reasons to persevere and attempt to overcome these difficulties.

REFERENCES

Ackerman, P. T., Dykman, R. A., & Peters, J. E. (1976). Hierarchical factor patterns on the WISC as related to areas of learning deficit. *Perceptual and Motor Skills, 42,* 583–615.

Ackerman, P. T., Dykman, R. A., & Peters, J. E. (1977). Learning-disabled boys as adolescents: Cognitive factors and achievement. *Journal of the American Academy of Child Psychiatry, 16,* 296–313.

Alexander, K. L., & Entwisle, D. R. (1988). Achievement in the first 2 years of school: Patterns and processes. *Monographs of the Society for Research in Child Development, 53*(2. Serial No. 218).

American Psychiatric Association. (1987). *Statistical manual of mental disorders* (3rd ed. rev.). Washington, DC: Author.

Blager, F. B. (1978). Response of emotionally disturbed children to auditory discrimination tests in quiet and noise. *Journal of Auditory Research, 18,* 221–227.

Blager, F. B., Zimet, S. G., & Farley, G. K. (1983). Auditory discrimination abilities of emotionally disturbed children in day psychiatric treatment: A replication study. *Journal of Auditory Research, 22,* 77–82.

Blatt, S. J., Chevron, E. S., Quinlan, D. M., & Wein, S. (1981). *The assessment of qualitative and structural dimensions of object representations.* New Haven: Yale University Press.

Blom, G. E., Farley, G. K., & Ekanger, C. (1973). A psychoeducational treatment program: Its characteristics and results. In G. E. Blom & G. K. Farley (Eds.), *Report on activities of the Day Care Center of the University of Colorado Medical Center to the Commonwealth Foundation.* Unpublished manuscript, University of Colorado Medical Center, Denver.

Bloom, R. B., Shea, R. J., & Eun, B. (1979). The Piers-Harris Scale: Norms for behaviorally disordered children. *Psychology in the Schools, 16,* 483–487.

Coopersmith, S. (1967). *The antecedents of self-esteem.* San Francisco: W. H. Freeman.

Corkey, C. L., & Zimet, S. G. (1987). Relationships with family and friends in young adulthood: A follow-up of children treated in a day hospital. *International Journal of Partial Hospitalization, 4,* 97–115.

Farley, G. K., & Zimet, S. G. (1987a). *Cortisol excretion of emotionally disturbed children in relationship to stress, anxiety, and competence.* Unpublished manuscript, University of Colorado Health Sciences Center, Denver.

Farley, G. K., & Zimet, S. G. (1987b). Can a five-minute verbal sample predict the response to day psychiatric treatment? *International Journal of Partial Hospitalization, 4,* 189–198.

Feshbach, N. D., & Feshbach, S. (1987). Affective processes and academic achievement. *Child Development, 58,* 1335–1347.

Foundation for Health Services Research. (1989, December). Mental health sessions at the AHSR/FHSR annual meeting focus on patient outcomes research. *Focus,* pp. 1–6.

Glasser, A. J., & Zimmerman, I. L. (1967). *Clinical interpretation of the Wechsler Intelligence Scale for Children (WISC).* New York: Grune & Stratton.

Goldman, R., Fristoe, M. S., & Woodcock, R. W. (1970). *Test of Auditory Discrimination.* Circle Pines, MN: American Guidance Service.

Gottschalk, L. A. (1974). A hope scale applicable to verbal samples. *Archives of General Psychiatry, 30,* 779–785.

Gottschalk, L. A. (1976). Children's speech as a source of data toward the measurement of psychological states. *Journal of Youth and Adolescence, 5,* 11–36.

Gottschalk, L. A. (1982). Manual of uses and applications of the Gottschalk-Gleser verbal behavior scales. *Research in Community Psychological and Psychiatric Behavior, 7,* 273–327.

Gottschalk, L. A., Uliana, R. L., & Hoigaard, J. C. (1979). Preliminary validation of a set of content analysis scales applicable to verbal samples for measuring the magnitude of psychological states in children. *Psychiatry Research, 1,* 71–82.

Group for the Advancement of Psychiatry. (1966). *Psychopathological disorders in childhood: Theoretical considerations and a proposed classification.* Washington, DC: American Psychiatric Association.

Harter, S. (1978). Perceived Competence Scale for Children manual: Form O. Denver: University of Denver.

Harter, S. (1982). The Perceived Competence Scale for Children. *Child Development, 53,* 87–97.

Heinicke, C. M., & Goldman, A. (1960). Research on psychotherapy with children: A review and suggestions for further study. *American Journal of Orthopsychiatry, 30,* 484–494.

Hollingshead, A. B., & Redlich, F. C. (1958). *Social class and mental illness.* New York: John Wiley & Sons.

Jackson, A. M., Farley, G. K., Zimet, S. G., & Gottman, J. M. (1979). Optimizing the WISC-R performance of low and high impulsive emotionally disturbed children. *Journal of Learning Disability, 12,* 622–625.

Jastak, J. F., & Jastak, S. R. (1965). *The Wide Range Achievement Test.* Wilmington: Guidance Associates of Delaware.

Jastak, J. F., & Jastak, S. R. (1978). *The Wide Range Achievement Test: Manual of instructions*. Wilmington, DE: Jastak Associates, Inc.

Kaufman, A. S. (1975). Factor analysis of the WISC-R at 11 age levels between 6½ and 16½ years. *Journal of Consulting and Clinical Psychology, 43*, 135–147.

LaVietes, R. L., Cohen, R., Reens, R., & Ronall, R. (1965). Day treatment center and school: Seven years experience. *American Journal of Orthopsychiatry, 35*, 160–169.

Lehrman, L. J., Sirluck, H., Black, B. J., & Glick, S. J. (1949). Success and failure of treatment of children in the child guidance clinics of the Jewish Board of Guardians. *Jewish Board of Guardians Research Monograph, 1*, 1–87.

Levitt, E. E. (1957). The results of psychotherapy with children: An evaluation. *Journal of Consulting and Clinical Psychology, 21*, 189–196.

Lufi, D., & Cohen, A. (1985). Using the WISC-R to identify attention deficit disorder. *Psychology in the Schools, 22*, 40–42.

Lufi, D., Cohen, A., & Parish-Plass, J. (1990). Identifying attention deficit hyperactive disorder with the WISC-R and the Stroop Color and Word Test. *Psychology in the Schools, 27*, 28–34.

Mead, G. H. (1934). *Mind, self and society.* Chicago: University of Chicago Press.

Miller, L. C. (1977a). *Louisville Behavior Checklist manual.* Los Angeles: Western Psychological Services.

Miller, L. C. (1977b). *School Behavior Checklist manual.* Los Angeles: Western Psychological Services.

Piers, E. V. (1969). *The Piers-Harris Children's Self-Concept Scale.* Nashville: Counselor Recordings and Tests.

Piers, E. V. (1972). Parent predictions of children's self-concepts. *Journal of Consulting and Clinical Psychology, 38*, 428–433.

Piers, E. V. (1984). *The Piers-Harris Children's Self-Concept Scale: Revised manual 1984.* Los Angeles: Western Psychological Services.

Porteus, S. E. (1942). *Qualitative performance in the Maze Test.* Vineland, NJ: Smith.

Prentice-Dunn, S., Wilson, D. R., & Lyman, R. D. (1981). Client factors related to outcome in a residential and day treatment program for children. *Journal of Clinical Child Psychology, 10*, 188–191.

Rogers, C. C. (1951). *Client-centered therapy.* Boston: Houghton Mifflin.

Sarason, S., Davidson, K., Lighthall, F., Waite, R., & Ruebush, B. (1960). *Anxiety in elementary school children.* New York: Wiley.

Silon, E. (1980). *Perceived competence, anxiety, and motivational orientation in educable mentally retarded children who are mainstreamed compared to those in self-contained classrooms.* Unpublished doctoral dissertation, University of Denver, Denver, Colorado.

Sullivan, H. S. (1953). *The interpersonal theory of psychiatry.* New York: Norton.

Wechsler, D. (1974). *Wechsler Intelligence Scale for Children—Revised.* New York: Psychological Corporation.

Wepman, J. M. (1973). *Auditory Discrimination Test.* Chicago: Language Research Associates.

Wolman, B. B. (1972). *Manual of child psychopathology.* New York: McGraw-Hill.

Wright, D. M., Moelis, I., & Pollack, L. J. (1976). The outcome of individual child psychotherapy: Increments at follow-up. *Journal of Child Psychology and Psychiatry, 17*, 275–285.

Zimet, G. D., Dahlem, N. W., Zimet, S. G., & Farley, G. K. (1988). The multidimensional scale of perceived social support. *Journal of Personality Assessment, 52*, 30–41.

Zimet, S. G., & Adler, S. S. (1990). Review of the use of abbreviated WISC-R forms with children with emotional disorders. *Journal of School Psychology, 28*, 133–146.

Zimet, S. G., & Farley, G. K. (1984). The self-concepts of children entering day psychiatric treatment. *Child Psychiatry and Human Development, 15*, 142–150.

Zimet, S. G., & Farley, G. K. (1985). Day treatment for children in the United States: Review article. *Journal of the American Academy of Child Psychiatry, 24,* 732–738.

Zimet, S. G., & Farley, G. K. (1986). Four perspectives on the competence and self-esteem of emotionally disturbed children beginning day treatment. *Journal of the American Academy of Child Psychiatry, 25,* 76–83.

Zimet, S. G., & Farley, G. K. (1987). How do emotionally disturbed children report their competencies and self-worth? *Journal of the American Academy of Child and Adolescent Psychiatry, 26,* 33–38.

Zimet, S. G., Farley, G. K., & Avitable, N. (1989). *Characteristics of children during and following day psychiatric treatment.* (Grant No. 1 R03 MH40993-01A1). Report to the Department of Health and Human Services, ADAMA Small Grant Program, National Institute of Mental Health. Rockville, MD: National Institute for Mental Health.

Zimet, S. G., Farley, G. K., & Dahlem, N. W. (1984). Behavior ratings of children in community schools and in day treatment. *International Journal of Partial Hospitalization, 2,* 199–208.

Zimet, S. G., Farley, G. K., & Dahlem, N. W. (1985). An abbreviated form of the WISC-R for use with emotionally disturbed children. *Psychology in the Schools, 22,* 19–22.

Zimet, S. G., Farley, G. K., Silver, J., Hebert, F. B., Robb, E. D., Ekanger, C., & Smith, D. (1980). Behavior and personality changes in emotionally disturbed children in a psychoeducational day treatment center. *Journal of The American Academy of Child Psychiatry, 19,* 240–256.

15

Relationships with Family and Friends in Young Adulthood
A Follow-Up of Children Treated in Our Day Hospital

CAROLINE L. CORKEY and SARA GOODMAN ZIMET

INTRODUCTION

Several investigators have reported that social relationship ratings of children by their peers or by their teachers have provided the best single predictor of social and emotional adjustment at later stages of life (Cass & Thomas, 1979; Cowen, Pederson, Babigan, Izzo, & Trost, 1973; Kagan & Moss, 1962). Children with negative ratings were more likely to have serious difficulties in school and at home than those with positive ratings. Furthermore, it has been reported by others that most emotionally disturbed children, in general, and those who are in day hospital settings, in particular, have problems in their interactions with their parents or other caregivers, their teachers, and/or their peers (Cass & Thomas, 1979; Zimet, Farley, & Dahlem, 1984).

According to object relations theory, these difficulties in interper-

From "Relationships with Family and Friends in Young Adulthood: A Follow-Up of Children Treated in a Day Hospital," by C. L. Corkey and S. G. Zimet, 1987, *International Journal of Partial Hospitalization, 4,* pp. 97–115. Copyright © 1987 by Plenum Publishing Corporation. Adapted by permission.

CAROLINE L. CORKEY and SARA GOODMAN ZIMET • The Day Care Center, Department of Psychiatry, University of Colorado Health Sciences Center, Denver, Colorado 80262.

sonal relationships may stem from serious disruptions in the infant and/or child–caregiver relationship (Bowlby, 1958, 1969; Spitz, 1965; Winnicott, 1960). The extent to which therapeutic interventions with children in a day hospital setting are likely to alter the risk of a negative outcome at later stages of life has received scant attention, however. Only six studies were published over a time span of approximately 40 years (1943 to 1981), and none looked at social relationships as a predictor outcome variable. Three of the studies examined children at the time they terminated day treatment (Goldfarb, Goldfarb, & Pollack, 1966; Prentice-Dunn, Wilson, & Lyman, 1981; Swan & Wood, 1975); two assessed children from 1 to 6 years after treatment had been terminated (Blom, Farley, & Ekanger, 1973; LaVietes, Cohen, Reens, & Ronall, 1965); and one examined the same group of children at three time points: termination, 3 to 6 months following termination, and 12 months after the first follow-up (Zimet, Farley, Silver, Hebert, Robb, Ekanger, & Smith, 1980). All the children at follow-up were under 18 years old.

The studies demonstrated that the majority of children during their pre, early, and late adolescence showed satisfactory adjustments in their community school placements. This finding also held for many of the children diagnosed at the beginning of treatment as schizophrenic (LaVietes *et al.,* 1965) and borderline (Blom *et al.,* 1973) as well as those in the moderately disturbed range. Furthermore, family instability rather than severity of psychopathology alone, was more likely than not to foretell a poor outcome (LaVietes *et al.,* 1965; Prentice-Dunn *et al.,* 1981). In addition, when comparing changes in behavior with progress in academic achievement, the greater improvement was made in the behavior domain, either at school or at home (Blom *et al.,* 1973; LaVietes *et al.,* 1965; Prentice-Dunn *et al.,* 1981; Zimet *et al.,* 1980). In effect, improvement in behavior and in academic achievement were found to be independent of one another (Prentice-Dunn *et al.,* 1981).

Although interpersonal relationships were not discussed directly in these studies, however, many of the questions answered by teachers and parents were concerned with the children's relationships with others. Therefore, the improvements reported on behavior ratings would appear to indicate that most children treated in day hospital settings did show positive changes in their interactions with the significant people in their lives.

With the absence of follow-up studies of young adults we are unable to determine, however, what the long-range adjustment might be at a time when new and increasingly difficult developmental tasks are being expected by the family and by society in general. The purpose of the present study, therefore, is to examine relationships with family and friends among a group of young adults who were identified in their middle-childhood years as emotionally disturbed. These relationships will be examined within a developmental object relations framework. We hypothesized that the majority of young adults studied will have achieved developmentally appropriate interpersonal relationships with parents, significant others, and friends. Because sex roles are differentiated along the lines of interpersonal relationships, we expected that the female young adults in this study will demonstrate a more mature stage of development than their male counterparts. Furthermore, we expect to find severity of the emotional disorder and age at the time of entry to day treatment to be significantly related to interpersonal relationships in young adulthood.

METHOD

Subjects

Potential Sample. The subjects of this study were 51 young adults between 18 and 25 years old. All had been enrolled during their middle childhood years in the day psychiatric hospital located in the Department of Psychiatry at the University of Colorado Health Sciences Center. A description of the subjects as to their gender, race, severity of childhood disorder, level of organicity at entry to day treatment, age at entry and termination from day hospital treatment, length of time in treatment, age at the time of the study, and length of time elapsed between termination and follow-up may be seen in Table 1. The methods used to determine severity of psychopathology and level of organicity are described below under Measures.

The theoretical orientation of the day hospital at the time the Potential Sample was enrolled was a psychodynamic one that utilized an interdisciplinary staff in the treatment of both children and parents. Children attended the program 6 hours a day, 5 days a week. Within that time structure, they were in classroom groups with both individualized and group experiences and were seen in individual psychotherapy twice a week. Their parents were seen once a week in family, conjoint, and/or individual therapy.

The Obtained and Lost Samples. The addresses for 37 (71%) of the 51 subjects were found and letters inviting their participation in the study were sent. Each letter was followed up by a phone call and appointments for a 2-hour interview were made with 22 (43%) of the 51 potential subjects. The 14 subjects whose family addresses had been found, were

Table 1. Characteristics of the Potential Sample Subjects

Characteristic	Potential sample ($N = 51$)	
Gender		
Male	36	(70.6%)
Female	15	(29.4%)
Race		
Black	6	(11.8%)
White	45	(88.2%)
Disorder		
Mild	20	(39.2%)
Moderate	20	(39.2%)
Severe	11	(21.6%)
Organicity		
None	10	(19.7%)
Minimal	22	(43.1%)
Moderate	16	(31.4%)
Severe	3	(5.8%)
Age		
At entry	9.8 years	
At termination	11.7 years	
At follow-up	22.1 years	
Time		
In treatment	1.9 years	
Termination to follow-up	11.7 years	

unavailable for a variety of reasons: (a) 5 lived outside of Colorado; (b) 2 had died, one of a kayak accident and the other by suicide; (c) 2 were unavailable for interviewing; and (d) 5 failed to show up for their appointments.

Table 2 presents information about the subjects who participated in the study (the Obtained Sample) and those who did not (the Lost Sample).

Comparisons were made between the two groups (OS vs. LS) using t-tests and chi-square tests. Our analyses indicated that there were no significant differences between them regarding entry age to day treatment, length of time in day treatment, and distribution by sex and by race. Significant differences, however, also were found that may help to account somewhat for the availability and willingness of those who participated in the study. For example, OS were older than LS at the time day treatment was terminated ($t = 2.42$, $p < .05$) and had a shorter time lapse between termination and follow-up ($t = 2.05$, $p < .05$). Thus, OS may have been more settled into an adult life pattern and may have felt more connected to the treatment center than LS. Furthermore, OS included significantly more subjects who were severely disturbed as chil-

Table 2. Characteristics of the Obtained and Lost Sample Subjects

Characteristic	Obtained sample (N = 22)		Lost sample (N = 29)	
Gender				
Male	14	(63.6%)	22	(75.9%)
Female	8	(36.4%)	7	(24.1%)
Race				
Black	1	(4.5%)	5	(17.2%)
White	21	(95.5%)	24	(82.8%)
Disorder				
Mild	5	(22.7%)	15	(51.7%)
Moderate	10	(45.5%)	10	(34.5%)
Severe	7	(31.8%)[a]	4	(13.8%)
Organicity				
None	2	(9.1%)	8	(27.6%)
Minimal	11	(50.0%)	11	(37.3%)
Moderate	6	(27.3%)	10	(34.4%)
Severe	3	(13.6%)[a]	0	(0.0%)
Age				
At entry	10.5 years		9.2 years	
At termination	12.5 years[b]		11.0 years	
At follow-up	22.0 years		22.0 years	
Time				
In treatment	2.1 years		1.8 years	
Termination to follow-up	11.2 years[b]		12.2 years	

[a]Test between Obtained and Lost samples is significant at the .002 level.
[b]Test between Obtained and Lost samples is significant at the .050 level.

dren than LS ($t = -3.33$, $p < .002$). In addition, all three of the subjects with severe organicity were in the OS group, which would tend to bias the findings against a positive outcome.

Procedures

As indicated appointments were made for one 2-hour interview when all data would be collected. A choice of a meeting place was given to all but two of the subjects, either at their home or in an office at the day psychiatric hospital where they had been in treatment as children. The two exceptions were interviewed in the institution where they were currently being treated because they had no other recourse. All signed an informed consent form prior to the interview and agreed to have the interview taped.

All interviews were conducted by the senior author who had no previous clinical knowledge of any subject at that time in order to reduce any bias that might influence the way questions were asked or the way answers were recorded.

The interview was divided into three parts. In the first part, the subject was presented with a list of life events derived from the Holmes-Rahe Social Readjustment Rating Scale (Holmes & Rahe, 1967). Then the subject was asked to identify those events that were relevant to their lives.

In the second part of the interview, the subject was asked questions from a semistructured interview that was developed by the senior author from instruments used by other investigators (Cass & Thomas, 1979; Vaillant, 1977) as well as from her many years of experience as a clinician. The questions were aimed at exploring the subjects' relationships with family members, friends, and significant others, their school and work status, and their physical and psychological health. The first draft of the interview was used with three young adult volunteers not connected with the study. Following this trial, the questionnaire was revised to its final form. If an event identified as relevant by the subject during the first part of the interview was not discussed during the semistructured interview, the interviewer reminded the subject of the event and asked questions about it. The interview was transcribed from the tapes and scored using the scales described under Measures.

The third and last part of the interview was spent administering the Multidimensional Scale of Perceived Social Support (MSPSS) (Zimet, Dahlem, Zimet, & Farley, 1988) also described here.

Measures

Perceptions of Parents

The Concept of the Object in Spontaneous Descriptions of Significant Figures Scale (Blatt, Chevron, Quinlan, & Wein, 1981). For purposes of brevity, we refer to this instrument as the Blatt Scale. The theoretical basis of the Blatt Scale was derived from Piagetian developmental psychology and object relations theory (Jacobson, 1964; Mahler, 1968; Piaget, 1954; Werner, 1957; Werner & Kaplan, 1963). It was developed using a sample of college sophomores, male and female, from two universities in the northeastern United States. Spontaneous descriptions of the subjects' mothers and fathers were collected from them, and a content analysis procedure was devised. For the purposes of this study, only Conceptual Level was scored for our subjects and this scale is described below:

Conceptual Level. Five developmental levels were identified, each describing a stage reached by a young adult in relationship with his or her parents. For scoring purposes, these levels (numbered 1, 3, 5, 7, and 9) were placed on the following 9-point scale:

1. Sensorimotor-Preoperational Level
2. High Sensorimotor-Preoperational Level
3. Concrete Perceptual Level
4. High Concrete Perceptual Level
5. External Iconic Level
6. High External Iconic Level
7. Internal Iconic Level
8. High Internal Iconic Level
9. Conceptual Level

The two levels believed to be appropriate to young adults are High Concrete Perceptual (a score of 4) and External Iconic (a score of 5). Both of these represent the achievement of a mature relationship with parents, where parents are increasingly recognized for their functions and attributes separate from the parenting ones. In effect, the separation–individuation process characterizing later adolescence and young adulthood is well on the way to being realized.

All references to and descriptions of each subject's father and mother were transcribed from the taped interviews and scored for conceptual level by a clinical psychology graduate student trained by Blatt and his associates.

Perceptions of Friends

The Friends Rating Scale (FRS). The FRS was developed by the senior author. Information given by the subject during the interview was rated on a 3-point scale, where 1 represented being very isolated with little to no contact with other people; 2 represented having casual social relationships within the context of a group; and 3 represented having meaningful and sustained social relationships with one or more close friends for more than 1 year.

The Multidimensional Scale of Perceived Social Support (MSPSS) (Zimet, Dahlem, Zimet, & Farley, 1988). At the time this study was carried out, the MSPSS consisted of 36 statements that describe the kind of support perceived by the subjects as being available to them from their family, friends, and significant others. The scale factored into three subscales of 12 items each, tapping the three sources of support aforementioned. It was administered during the third part of the interview. After a statement was read to the subject, he or she was asked to select an answer from a 7-point scale. The answers ranged from "Very Strongly Agree"

Table 3. Weighted Means for Diagnostic Categories

Diagnostic category	Weighted mean
Psychotic	11.00
Delinquent	9.67
Schizoid	9.00
Aggressive	6.70
Somatic	6.33
Depressed	6.00
Obsessive-compulsive	5.00
Social withdrawal	4.00
Uncommunicative	3.67
Hyperactive	2.50

with a value of 7 (high score) to "Very Strongly Disagree" with a value of 1 (low score). Scores were obtained for each of the three subscales by the senior author, using a scoring key provided with the scale.

Severity of Disturbance. A list of 11 diagnostic categories was compiled by the senior author and the director of the day hospital. The list was based on the categories defined in the Child Behavior Checklist (Achenbach, 1983) and on the director's experience in diagnosing the children in the day hospital. The 11 categories were then ranked from most severe psychopathology to least severe psychopathology by each of three clinicians. A weighted mean was thus obtained for each diagnostic category. "Psychotic" received the highest mean, whereas "Hyperactive" received the lowest mean. The weighted means for all 11 diagnostic categories may be seen in Table 3.

An appraisal of psychopathology at the time a subject entered the day psychiatric hospital was made, *post hoc,* by the child psychiatrist who was the director at the day hospital. As each subject's treatment chart was reviewed, either a "yes" or "no" was written next to each of the 11 categories. The weighted means of all "yes" scores were added together. The groups' total scores were then divided into three severity groups: (a) those representing mild psychopathology (scores to 10.9); (b) those representing moderate psychopathology (scores between 11 and 20); and (c) those representing severe psychopathology (scores between 20.1 and 50).

Level of Organicity. The center's director also determined from *post hoc* chart review the level of organicity for each subject when he or she entered the day psychiatric hospital. This was done using a 4-point classification system, with 1 representing "No Neurological Signs Present" and 4 representing "Severe Organicity."

The neurological signs included motor incoordination, hyper-kinesis, perceptual dysfunction, poor concentration, and deficiency in verbal skills. Pathognomonic evidence from past records was also considered. Minimal organicity was defined as having one to two of the neurological signs; moderate organicity required three to five of the neurological signs; and severe organicity involved five of the neurological signs and/or pathognomonic evidence from a neurological examination or history.

Age at Entry. Subjects were assigned to the following four age groups:

Group   I: (N = 5) 5.9 years to 9.5 years.
Group II: (N = 5) 9.6 years to 10.7 years.
Group III: (N = 7) 10.8 years to 11.5 years.
Group IV: (N = 5) 11.6 years to 14.5 years.

All analyses were done using these groupings.

Data Analysis

The Blatt standardization sample (BSS) was within the same age range as the young adults in the present study (OS). Therefore, OS scores were compared with BSS scores. Comparisons between and within subject groups were done using t-tests. When the test for homogeneity of variances was significant, the t-test using different estimates of degrees of freedom was employed.

Relationships between variables were examined using a one-way analysis of variance, chi-square tests, and Pearson product moment correlation coefficients.

FINDINGS

The Obtained Sample as Young Adults

The majority of the Obtained Sample (16 or 72.7%) were single. This proportion includes 3 who were divorced. The remaining 6 (27.3%) were married, one by common law.

Living arrangements were evenly divided among those living with a significant other (either married, in a common-law relationship, or unmarried) (7 or 31.8%), those living with parents (8 or 36.4%), and those living in group situations (7 or 31.8%). Of this latter group, 4 were in one of the following treatment settings: (a) a chronic psychiatric inpatient ward; (b) a vocational rehabilitation program of an adult day psychiatric hospital; (c) a drug treatment center; and (d) an outpatient alcohol treatment program.

Half the subjects (11) were either enrolled in or graduated from high school; slightly over one-third ($N = 8$) had left high school without graduating; and 3 had gone on to college (13.6%).

Most of the young adults (17 or 77.3%) were employed on either a part-time or full-time basis. Of the 5 who were unemployed (22.7%), 3 were in residential treatment, one was taking care of her new baby at home, and one was living in his parents' home.

Perception of Parents

The Blatt Scale

Conceptual Level and Gender. Table 4 presents the Conceptual Level mean scores and standard deviations for each pair of comparisons made.

OS Females vs. OS Males. As we predicted, both females and males in the Obtained Sample were at appropriate developmental Conceptual Levels for young adults as regards their relationships with mothers (External Iconic and Concrete Perceptual Level respectively) and with fathers (both External Iconic). They described both parents as being independent of themselves. Males' Conceptual Level scores for mothers, however, were significantly lower than those obtained by females ($t(20) = 2.73$, $p < .01$). In effect, OS females achieved a more advanced developmental level in their relationships with mothers than had their male counterparts. There were no sex differences as regards relationships with fathers.

Table 4. Comparisons of Conceptual Level Scores of Females (F) and Males (M) in the Obtained Sample (OS) and in Blatt's Standardization Sample (BSS)

	Conceptual level (mothers)		Conceptual level (fathers)	
	M	SD	M	SD
OS females vs.	5.00[a]	1.31	4.98	1.55
OS males	3.64	1.01	4.07	1.39
OS females vs.	5.00	1.31	4.83	1.55
BSS females	4.84	1.64	4.83	1.71
OS males vs.	3.64[a]	1.01	4.07	1.39
BSS males	4.82	1.37	4.96	1.40

[a] $p < .01$.

Jane, who achieved an appropriate developmental level, used some of the following sentences to describe her mother: "My mother worked as a secretary and now [is] married and so [her] income has gone up. I have been closest to my mother. Mother is reserving judgment about me. I think on the whole she thinks things are progressing well. I am not disturbed anymore. That's what they would say; I am not emotionally disturbed. I am not so antisocial and I am not so destructive . . . my mother . . . we enjoy almost anything we do together. We just like each other. We always see each other. We just like each other."

Leo described his mother and stepmother in more concrete terms. "My mother left when I was 1½. Father went through a divorce since Day Care. . . . I was 12 or 13 when they divorced [he and my stepmother]. It didn't affect me the way it could. I didn't have the best relationship with my stepmother. . . . She would resent [my] personal achievement. . . . I was told by my stepmother I would never make it [in the Army]; I wasn't cut out [to succeed] . . . [but] the farther I go the more I achieve."

OS Females vs. BSS Females. Both female groups achieved Conceptual Level scores in the External Iconic range (Ms = 5.00 and 4.84 respectively), indicating that those young adults who had been in day psychiatric treatment as children did not differ significantly from the Blatt Scale's standardization sample in the descriptions of relationships with either parent.

OS Males vs. BSS Males. In their descriptions of mothers, these two groups of young adults differed significantly in their Conceptual Level scores (t (52) = 2.94, p < .01). Males who had been in day psychiatric treatment as children, although being at an appropriate developmental level (Concrete Perceptual), had significantly lower scores than the college males (External Iconic). As with their female counterparts, both groups of males attained Conceptual Level scores within the External Iconic range in their descriptions of fathers.

Conceptual Level and Age at Entry. Moderately strong inverse relationships were found between entry age and Conceptual Level scores on the Blatt Scale (Mother and Father rs = −.58, p < .005 and −.48, p < .02 respectively). The earlier the entry age into day hospital treatment, the higher the developmental level of young adults in the descriptions of their relationships with both parents.

Conceptual Level and Severity of Psychopathology at Entry. Although we found no significant differences between Conceptual Level scores in young adulthood and severity of emotional disorders in childhood, a trend was noted (F 2,7 (19) = 3.17, p < .06). Those in the mildly severe group had the highest Conceptual Level scores, and those in the most severe group had the lowest Conceptual Level scores.

Perception of Friends

Friends Rating Scale

Gender. The majority of subjects (15 or 68.2%) indicated that they had sustained friendships, those lasting for 1 or more years; 13% ($N = 3$) stated that they had casual friendships only. All of the females and 71% of the males had ratings within these first two categories. The remaining four subjects (18.2%), all males, made up the isolated group who had little or no contact with people outside their families. In effect, the prediction that most of the young adults would have achieved developmentally appropriate interpersonal relationships with friends was supported.

Severity of Psychopathology. Significant differences were found between the proportion of subjects with Mild, Moderate, and Severe psychopathology in childhood and the quality of their friendships as young adults (χ^2 (4) = 22, $p < .02$). All of the subjects in the Mild psychopathology group ($N = 5$) and 8 of the 10 in the Moderate group described their friendships as being meaningful and long-standing ones. Over half of the subjects in the severely disturbed group (4 of the 7) described themselves as having no friendships. Of further interest, however, is that of the remaining 3 subjects diagnosed in childhood as severely disturbed, 2 indicated that they currently had sustained relationships and one had casual relationships.

> Joan is an interesting example of a young woman who had been diagnosed as autistic as a child but who achieved sustained relationships as a young adult. She illustrated her ability to relate with a simple but sensitive picture of her mother. She said of her mother, "She is optimistic; she is hardworking. . . . She got her M.A. in about 1979, I guess . . . then she was looking for a job. . . . When she works, she gets totally involved in her work. . . . We are very close, really close. I think it is because we are opposites. I feel I am more like my Dad and she is more social. And she is more of a warm person than I am. Always, throughout my life, she has been a great help. I always sympathize with her when there is a problem and she confides in me. I told her just about all my problems."

Perceptions of Family and Friends

Multidimensional Scale of Perceived Social Support (MSPSS)

Gender. The mean scores for males and females were similar across the three factors tapped by this scale, perceived support from Family (5.11 and 5.22 respectively), from Friends (5.04 and 5.59 respectively), and from Significant Others (5.78 and 5.62 respectively). These data indicated that both male and female young adult subjects felt they could depend on the people from their immediate social network for the support they needed.

Age at Entry. We found a moderate nonsignificant inverse relationship between entry age and two scales of the MSPSS: perceptions of support from Friends and from Significant Others ($rs = -.35$). Age, in effect, contributed only 12% to the unexplained variance of perceived support from Friends and from Significant Others.

Severity of Psychopathology at Entry. We found no significant differences among the three severity groups and the three scales of the MSPSS. How these young adults viewed their support network appeared to be unrelated to the level of their psychopathology as children.

Relationships among Measures

The Blatt Scale, the Multidimensional Scale of Perceived Social Support, and the Friends Rating Scale. The only strong relationship we found was between the Friends Rating Scale and the Friends Scale of the MSPSS ($r = .71$, $p < .001$). Young adults who described themselves as having long-term relationships were also likely to perceive their friends as a source of support.

Moderate positive relationships were demonstrated in all but one of the comparisons made between mothers' and fathers' Conceptual Level scores of the Blatt Scale and MSPSS and FRS scores. Correlations ranged from .40 to .55 with the one exception being a .21 correlation between perceived support from Family and mothers' Conceptual Level scores. In general, then, these findings indicate that young adults who are at a higher developmental level in their relationships with both parents have a good likelihood of experiencing meaningful and sustained relationships with friends as well as support from the people within their social network.

In general, each measure used in this study was tapping both similar and different facets of interpersonal relationships.

DISCUSSION

The majority of female and male young adults in this study appeared to be at appropriate developmental levels in their relationships with parents, with significant others, and with friends. In addition, most of them felt that they had recourse to a substantial level of support from the significant people in their lives. Although most achieved appropriate levels of separation and individuation from mothers and fathers, female young adults demonstrated a more mature level of development in relationships with mothers than did their male counterparts (External Iconic vs. Concrete Perceptual). This sex difference did not show up in relationships with fathers, where both males and females scored at the External Iconic Level. Neither did it show up in the quality of friendships nor in perceptions of support from the significant people in their lives. Consequently, the prediction that females in this study would demonstrate a more mature stage of development than their male counterparts in their descriptions of their relationships with the significant people in their lives was not strongly substantiated. One possible explanation for the sex differences found on the Conceptual Level Scale with mothers may relate to the preponderance of males in the present study who were diagnosed in childhood as having high levels of severe psychopathology and organicity. These conditions may have extended the period of dependency for sons on mothers, who were their primary caretakers, and delayed, somewhat, the process of breaking away and being on their own. Because no sex differences were found on this dimension in the Blatt Standardization Sample but was seen in the comparison of OS and BSS males (Concrete Perceptual vs. External Iconic), this explanation would appear to be a feasible one.

Severity of diagnosis in childhood appeared to exert an influence on interpersonal relationships in young adulthood. The young adults described were primarily those who were diagnosed in childhood as mildly or moderately emotionally disturbed ($N = 15$). All but one described their interpersonal relationships in the predicted direction. Conversely, all but one of the subjects in the most severely disordered group ($N = 7$) showed the worst prognosis for interpersonal relationships in adulthood. As indicated, they tended to have the lowest Conceptual Level scores in relationships with mothers, and they were more likely to be social isolates. These findings would seem to raise questions regarding the need to review treatment goals and plans for severely disordered children and their families. LaVietes *et al.* (1965) and Goldfarb *et al.* (1966) both raised this issue as regards the stability of the home environment for these children. In effect, both studies questioned the advisability of day psychiatric placement for these most severely disordered children from emotionally unstable families. On the other hand, day hospital treatment can provide a stable environment in a treatment milieu where the family's ability to provide a healthy environment for the child can be evaluated. The outcome of the evaluation may result in placement outside the child's home or continued efforts to work with the family and the child together in the day treatment setting.

The issue of the emotional status of the family was not examined in the present study because the information was not recorded on the subjects' clinical charts at the time they were in day treatment, however prospective studies should take this factor into account.

In a review of studies that examined the influence of severity of psychopathology in childhood on later adjustment, Gelfand and Peterson (1985) found that children rarely overcame such problems as conduct disorders, autism, psychoses, underachievement, and rejection by peers. Instead, the presence of these problems was likely to foreshadow adult maladjustment. In this population of young adults who had received intensive milieu therapy in their middle childhood years, most had conduct disorders, were underachievers, and were rejected by peers, and a smaller proportion were seen as schizophrenic, psychotic, and borderline. As young adults, however, most were functioning at a level of development appropriate for their stage in life as regards their relationships with others.

As predicted, early age at entry to day treatment appeared to be significantly related to more mature perceptions of relationships with parents in young adulthood. These findings lend support to results from two other studies that examined the relationship of age to outcome of day hospital treatment and to which we referred earlier in this chapter. Blom and his associates (1973) found age to be the only variable demonstrating significant discriminatory power. Young children were more likely to have better outcome ratings than older children. Similarly, Prentice-Dunn and his colleagues (1981) found that children who showed the most positive behavioral changes were youngest when day psychiatric treatment was begun.

The extent to which age and severity of psychopathology at entry interacted may account somewhat for this finding. A *post hoc* analysis indicated that these two variables were significantly associated ($p < .02$) in the present study. In effect, the young adults who had entered day treatment at an early age were less severely disturbed than those who entered day treatment when they were older. We think it may be that the community and parents of these younger children were more attuned to their needs and sought help before the problems became more severe. This explanation, in turn, may shed some light on the finding that children entering day treatment at an earlier age had more mature relationships with their parents than did children entering at a later age. On the other hand, such an explanation precludes the notion that the older children had been in another treatment setting prior to admission to day hospital treatment. We do not know whether the most severely disturbed group were in other treatment settings prior to entering the day hospital because this information was not systematically recorded in their clinical charts. Nevertheless, we think that age at entry to day hospital treatment is probably not a reliable indicator of age at entry into the mental health service system.

Those young adults who were in the Severe Group as children also included those who had high levels of organic involvement. As discussed earlier, we expected, therefore, that children diagnosed as severely disturbed would be more likely to remain in a dependent relationship with their parents and other caregivers than would those diagnosed with a Mild level of psychopathology and Low level of organicity. The finding, therefore, that young adults diagnosed as mildly disturbed in childhood were at a higher developmental level in relationships with parents than those in the Severe diagnostic group is not entirely surprising. In future prospective follow-up studies, both age and severity (psychopathology and organicity) at entry to day hospital treatment should be examined.

An ideal design for an outcome study would be to randomly assign subjects to treatment (inpatient, day hospital, and outpatient) and no-treatment groups. Ethical and legal issues arise, however, regarding this approach of withholding treatment or assigning patients to a treatment modality randomly. Furthermore, there is little likelihood that the children's parents would accept this arrangement. The absence of a control group was handled partially (on the Blatt Scale only) by using the young adults on which the Blatt Scale was developed as a normative population with which to be compared.

Some of the other problems inherent in long-term follow-up studies that were experienced in this investigation included locating and recruiting subjects. Many had moved away and left no forwarding address. Furthermore, the increasing public concerns about confidentiality provided limited access to school, hospital, and court records. Thus there is some concern regarding the generalizability of these findings to the total sample of children treated in the specific day hospital from which the subjects were drawn as well as to young adults who had been treated in other day hospital settings with similar therapeutic orientations.

Although there was a relatively high attrition rate, we were nevertheless able to compare the Lost and Obtained Samples on a number of variables that had been systematically recorded on all of their clinical charts and on *post hoc* diagnoses of psychopathology and organicity at entry to day hospital treatment. The groups did not differ on basic demographic characteristics listed on their charts, suggesting that the Obtained Sample is generally representative of the total sample from which it was drawn. They did differ, however, on the *post hoc* assessments done. The more severely disturbed and organically impaired were over-represented in the Obtained Sample. They also tended to stand apart from the other children lending credibility to the *post hoc* ratings of severity levels. Because of the findings regarding severity, we recommend that assessments made at the time day treatment began be systematically recorded in order to provide more reliable information on this dimension in future follow-up studies.

The only source of information on interpersonal relationships was the subjects themselves, not their parents, not their friends, not their significant others. It is difficult for us to know, therefore, if there would have been large discrepancies among the raters. Although these discrepancies would not necessarily invalidate the perspectives presented by the young adults studied, they might provide a more realistic description of the relationships among the significant people in their lives.

CONCLUSIONS

Keeping in mind the qualifications mentioned, the findings from the present investigation upheld the hypothesis that the majority of young adults studied would be at developmentally appropriate levels in their interpersonal relationships with parents, friends, and significant others. The expectation that females would be at a more mature level than males because of sex role socialization patterns was not strongly supported, however. Children beginning day hospital treatment at an earlier age, who were considered mild in the severity of their disorder and low in level of organicity, appeared to manage the separation–individuation process better as young adults than children who were older, more severely disturbed, and with higher levels of organicity. Furthermore, there were more similarities than differences between the young adults who were considered to be at high risk for psychopathology in adulthood and young adults who were among the Blatt standardization sample. These findings, we believe, appear to extend the results discussed earlier of follow-up studies of children under 18 years old and suggest that intensive psychodynamically oriented milieu day treatment during the middle childhood years may be a therapeutic intervention powerful enough to favorably influence interpersonal relationships in young adulthood.

ACKNOWLEDGMENTS

This chapter is based on research conducted by the first author in partial fulfillment of the Ph.D. requirements of Smith College School of Social Work. Some of the findings were presented at the First National

Conference on Child and Adolescent Day Treatment, Pasadena, California, May 1987. She gratefully acknowledges the assistance of Gordon K. Farley, Claire Purcell, and Robert Harmon, of the University of Colorado Health Sciences Center, in applying their clinical expertise to the diagnosis, coding, and rating of the data; Nanci Avitable, of the University of Colorado Health Sciences Center, and Gregory Zimet, of Case Western Reserve University, for their excellent consultation regarding the statistical analyses; Charlie Wilbur, of Yale University, for scoring the verbal samples; Roger Miller and Natalie Hill, of Smith College, for their invaluable suggestions in designing and carrying out this study; and Elizabeth Root and Nina Gasiorowicz, of Smith College, for their comments on earlier drafts of this chapter.

REFERENCES

Achenbach, T. M. (1983). *Manual For The Child Behavior Checklist and revised Child Behavior Profile*. Burlington, VT: University Associates in Psychiatry.

Blatt, S. J., Chevron, E. S., Quinlan, D. M., & Wein, S. (1981). *The assessment of qualitative and structural dimensions of object representations*. New Haven: Yale University Press.

Blom, G. E., Farley, G. K., & Ekanger, C. (1973). A psychoeducational treatment program: Its characteristics and results. In G. E. Blom & G. K. Farley (Eds.), *Report on activities of the Day Care Center of the University of Colorado Medical Center to the Commonwealth Foundation*. Unpublished manuscript, University of Colorado Medical Center, Department of Psychiatry.

Bowlby, J. (1958). The nature of the child's tie to his mother. *International Journal of Psychoanalysis, 39,* 350–373.

Bowlby, J. (1969). *Attachment and loss* (Vol. 1). New York: Basic Books.

Cass, L. M., & Thomas, C. B. (1979). *Childhood pathology and later adjustment*. New York: John Wiley & Sons.

Cowen, E. L., Pederson, R., Babigan, H., Izzo, L. D., & Trost, M. A. (1973). Follow-up of early detected vulnerable children. *Journal of Consulting and Clinical Psychology, 41,* 438–446.

Gelfand, D. M., & Peterson, L. (1985). *Child development and psychopathology*. Beverly Hills: Sage Publications.

Goldfarb, W., Goldfarb, N., & Pollack, R. C. (1966). Treatment of childhood schizophrenics. *Archives of General Psychiatry, 14,* 114–128.

Holmes, T. H., & Rahe, R. H. (1967). The Social Readjustment Rating Scale. *Journal of Psychosomatic Research, 11,* 213–218.

Jacobson, E. (1964). *The self and the object world*. New York: International Universities Press.

Kagan, J., & Moss, H. R. (1962). *Birth to maturity*. New York: John Wiley & Sons.

LaVietes, R. L., Cohen, R., Reens, R., & Ronall, A. (1965). Day treatment center and school: Seven years experience. *American Journal of Orthopsychiatry, 35,* 160–169.

Mahler, M. S. (1968). On the concepts of symbiosis and separation-individuation. In M. S. Mahler & M. Furer (Eds.), *On human symbiosis and the vicissitudes of individuation* (pp. 7–31). New York: International Universities Press.

Piaget, J. (1954). *The construction of reality in the child*. New York: Basic Books.

Prentice-Dunn, S., Wilson, D. R., & Lyman, R. D. (1981). Client factors related to outcome in a residential and day treatment program for children. *Journal of Clinical Child Psychology, 10,* 188–191.

Spitz, R. A. (1965). *The first year of life.* New York: International Universities Press.

Swan, W. W., & Wood, M. M. (1975). Making decisions about treatment. In M. M. Wood (Ed.), *Developmental therapy.* Austin, TX: Pro-ed.

Vaillant, G. E. (1977). *Adaptation to life.* Boston: Little, Brown.

Werner, H. (1957). *Comparative psychology of mental development* (rev. ed.). New York: International Universities Press.

Werner, H., & Kaplan, B. (1963). *Symbol formation: An organismic-developmental approach to language and the expression of thought.* New York: John Wiley & Sons.

Winnicott, D. W. (1960). The theory of the parent-infant relationship. *International Journal of Psychoanalysis, 41,* 585–595.

Zimet, G. D., Dahlem, N. W., Zimet, S. G., & Farley, G. K. (1988). The multidimensional scale of perceived social support. *Journal of Personality Assessment, 52,* 30–41.

Zimet, S. G., Farley, G. K., Silver, J., Hebert, F. B., Robb, E. D., Ekanger, C., & Smith, D. (1980). Behavior and personality changes in emotionally disturbed children enrolled in a psychoeducational day treatment center. *Journal of the American Academy of Child Psychiatry, 19,* 240–252.

Zimet, S. G., Farley, G. K., & Dahlem, N. W. (1984). Behavior ratings of children in community schools and in day treatment. *International Journal of Partial Hospitalization, 2,* 199–208.

Index